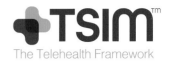

T0206796

TSIM: The Telehealth Framework
A comprehensive guide to telehealth implementation and optimization

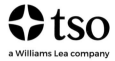

Published by TSO (The Stationery Office Limited) ("Publisher"),
a part of Williams Lea, and available from:

Online: www.tsoshop.co.uk

Mail, Telephone, Fax & E-mail:
TSO
PO Box 29, Norwich, NR3 1GN
Telephone orders/General enquiries: 0333 202 5070
Fax orders: 0333 202 5080
E-mail: customer.services@tso.co.uk
Textphone: 0333 202 5077

ISBN 9780117092969

Printed in the United Kingdom for The Stationery Office
J003806414 c5 09/21

Contents

Acknowledgements

Shawn Valenta, *Editor*

Dee Ford, *Associate Editor*

Contributors

Shawn Valenta RRT, MHA. Vice President of Healthcare Cloud – Clinical Services, Wellpath; Affiliate Faculty, Medical University of South Carolina

Dee W. Ford MD, MCSR. Division Director and Professor of Pulmonary and Critical Care Medicine, Medical University of South Carolina; Program Director, National Telehealth Center of Excellence, Medical University of South Carolina

Emily Warr MSN, RN. Administrator for Telehealth, Medical University of South Carolina

James T. McElligott MD, MSCR. Executive Medical Director for Telehealth, Medical University of South Carolina; Associate Professor in the Division of General Paediatrics, Medical University of South Carolina Children's Hospital

Jillian Harvey MPH, PhD. Associate Professor in Healthcare Leadership and Management, Medical University of South Carolina; Director for the Doctor of Health Administration Division, Medical University of South Carolina

Kathryn King MD, MHS. Associate Executive Medical Director, Center for Telehealth, Medical University of South Carolina; Associate Program Director for the National Telehealth Center of Excellence, Medical University of South Carolina.

The contributors would like to thank the following people from MUSC whose input was indispensable to this publication: Ellen Debenham, Jessica Dustman, Meghan Glanville, Emily Sederstrom, Bryna Rickett, and Tasia Walsh.

Reviewers

We kindly thank those who took part in the review process:

Najib Ben Brahim, PhD. CEO, Ignis Health

Bonnie Bernard, BSN, RN, CCHP. IT Director of Telehealth, Wellpath

Linda Branagan, PhD. Director, Telehealth Programs, University of California, San Francisco

Kyle Brewer. Telehealth Administrator, University of Mississippi Medical Center

Julie Hall-Barrow, EdD, FATA. Senior Vice President, Network Development and Innovation, Children's Health

Kristi Henderson, DNP, NP-C, FAAN. Senior Vice President, Center for Digital Health & Innovation, Optum Health; CEO, MedExpress

Alan Pitt, MD. Professor, Neuroradiology, Barrow Neurological Institute; Co-founder, Vitalchat

Foreword

TSIM: A framework for change

In March 2020, the world faced an existential threat. The global pandemic that was caused by a virus brought everything to a screeching halt. COVID-19 changed the paradigms we had grown accustomed to. In order for an organization to survive, regardless of product or service, it had no choice but to change with immediacy, and this was often done with limited hindsight or foresight. Healthcare was one area that impacted all of us. Individuals in need of routine medical care and the medical personnel providing this care had to communicate mostly via telemedicine, telehealth, or not at all – which was, and remains, a challenge for many.

Throughout the 20th century, the idea of providing healthcare remotely over some distance has been like a rollercoaster at an amusement park. Even though the technology was slowly changing, the idea of changing anything was even slower. Government funding for research projects and testbeds ramped up then declined, only to ramp up and decline again. This cycle was finally broken at the turn of the 21st century, primarily due to innovation in computing and telecommunications. Tempered by the inherent need in space exploration and on the battlefield, and the insatiable desire to reduce cost and improve care, telemedicine and telehealth began to be more acceptable as a mode of healthcare delivery. Yet, it remained elusive for many, simply because of attitude, awareness, and a lack of standard program development and operations.

Telehealth has seen unprecedented growth as a direct result of the global pandemic, with rapid increase in the integration and adoption of telehealth in clinical settings worldwide. What took decades to become accepted practice literally changed overnight. Across the landscape of America's academic health centers, several ecosystems have established themselves as true leaders. The Medical University of South Carolina (MUSC) is one such example. It has embraced change in an effort to address the healthcare needs across its state and region.

MUSC began its telehealth journey in 2005 with an innovative endeavor to improve maternal fetal health in a rural, medically underserved region of the state. After several years of gaining traction and experience with a wide variety of telehealth applications, the program was recognized by the American Telemedicine Association in 2019 as a leading program in the US. In addition, MUSC is one of only two HRSA-designated National Telehealth Centers of Excellence in the US. The Telehealth Service Implementation Model (TSIM) framework developed by MUSC, and now adopted by organizations across the US, supports health systems in developing, implementing, and maintaining a telehealth solution.

The TSIM framework was created using a foundation of telehealth best practices and has continued to mature through MUSC's vast experience in telehealth service development and implementation. TSIM utilizes common terminology for the development of services and provides standardized processes to address specific telehealth issues. TSIM is comprised of six phases:

- Pipeline (which flows into the broader TSIM structure)
- Strategy
- Development
- Implementation
- Operations
- Continuous Quality Improvement.

Each phase has associated tasks that must be reviewed and, if applicable, completed before a service advances to the next phase.

These six stages of the TSIM framework serve as a roadmap to successfully develop, implement, and sustain telehealth services. TSIM provides an architecture and terminology to enhance the clinical, technical, and administrative collaboration required to successfully establish and provide effective telehealth services that are integrated into the traditional care delivery system, and are of high utility to both patient and provider. In addition, it provides strategic principles and philosophies that aid in redesigning care delivery (not simply using video to replicate the existing inefficiencies and in-person processes). TSIM is currently being adopted by healthcare organizations across the US, helping to simplify the complexities of telehealth service development, implementation, and management.

This unique publication brings together information and guidance to enlighten the reader with knowledge that can be put to use immediately. TSIM provides telehealth teams, both clinical and technical, with a systematic approach and common language to proactively recognize their strengths, weaknesses, and gaps in service development, implementation, and management. The TSIM model provides an excellent resource for all involved in developing and deploying telemedicine and telehealth.

Charles R. Doarn, MBA, FATA, FAsMA

Research Professor, Department of Environmental and Public Health Sciences
MPH Program Director, College of Medicine, University of Cincinnati
Director, UC Space Research Institute for Discovery and Exploration
Special Assistant to the NASA Chief Health and Medical Officer

Preface

Telehealth is rapidly advancing along the diffusion-of-innovation curve. Early innovators, such as Dr. Jay Sanders, Charles Doarn, and Dr. Rashid Bashur, identified telehealth service development and implementation challenges, and began illuminating a pathway forward. Subsequent innovators, such as the Medical University of South Carolina (MUSC), advanced telehealth through a focus on clinical strategy and a vision to apply telehealth to improve the efficiency and effectiveness of patient care.

The public health emergency caused by the COVID-19 pandemic resulted in such a pervasive uptake of telehealth that telehealth is now solidly in the early-majority phase of the adoption curve. What the field is lacking is a comprehensive and practical "how to" guide for successful telehealth service development, implementation, and sustainment. TSIM is that guide and has simplified the complexities of telehealth implementation and optimization. TSIM will take users from an initial telehealth idea to successful program sustainment by leading them through the development of a strategy-driven telehealth approach, structured program development pathways, outcomes-driven evaluation, financial sustainability, and ongoing operations.

Our goal is that the TSIM framework will catalyze a new renaissance in digital health adoption, moving more service ideas towards the journey to scale. It is time to apply telehealth to forge new models of healthcare delivery and a system that delivers high-quality, cost-effective, and equitable care.

Shawn Valenta
Editor

1 | Overview

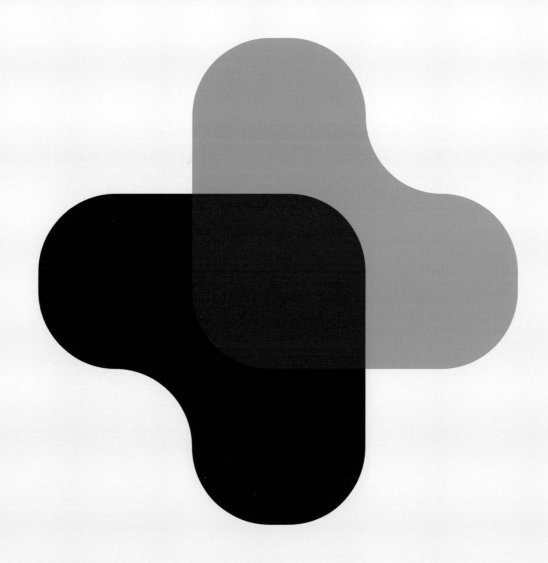

1.1 Introduction

The United States healthcare industry is in the midst of a digital transformation, striving to reform, strengthen, and modernize the nation's healthcare system.[1] The US spends more money per capita on healthcare than any other country.[2] When reviewing healthcare expenditures as a percentage of the gross domestic product (GDP), it can be seen that the US spends nearly twice as much as other similar nations. In addition, it has fewer practicing physicians as a percentage of the population, which may be driving fewer physician visits. Simultaneously, the US has among the highest rates of obesity and chronic disease burden. Fueled by increased healthcare spending, provider shortages, and an aging population, a shift towards more efficient, effective care is imperative.

The United States Health Resources & Services Administration (HRSA) defines *telehealth* as "the use of electronic information and telecommunication technologies to support long-distance clinical health care, patient and professional health-related education, public health, and health administration."[3] Telehealth has been identified as an effective tool to address many of the challenges of the US healthcare system, including reducing cost, increasing access, and improving quality.[4]

As record-setting investments further catalyze the development of telehealth solutions, many healthcare providers are expected to move forward in their digital transformation efforts. Unfortunately, barriers to telehealth development and implementation have historically frustrated healthcare providers, and continue to do so.[5] Hospitals and physician practices, especially those in rural regions, that do not adapt to the evolving healthcare environment and adopt telehealth capabilities will likely not survive in their present forms. Without a systematic telehealth implementation approach, healthcare providers should expect continued frustrations and varied results.

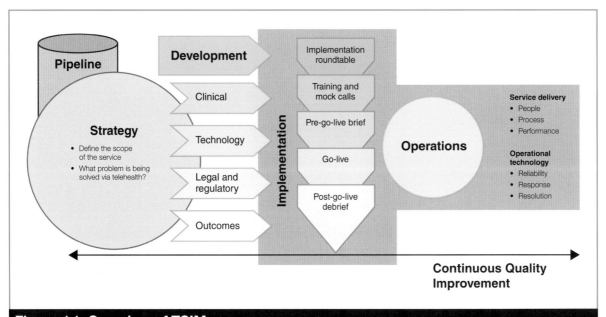

Figure 1.1 Overview of TSIM

This introduction to the Telehealth Service Implementation Model (TSIM) is intended to support health systems and providers on their journey to advance the adoption of telehealth development and implementation (see Figure 1.1). TSIM is a guiding framework that has evolved out of the extensive telehealth experience at the Medical University of South Carolina (MUSC), one of only two HRSA-designated National Telehealth Centers of Excellence in the US.

The TSIM framework was created with a foundation of telehealth best practices, and has continued to mature through MUSC's vast experience in telehealth service development and implementation. TSIM establishes common terminology for the development of services and provides standardized processes to address specific telehealth issues. It includes six phases:

- Pipeline (which flows into the broader TSIM structure)
- Strategy
- Development
- Implementation
- Operations
- Continuous Quality Improvement.

Each phase has associated tasks that must be reviewed and, if applicable, completed before a service advances to the next phase. TSIM provides telehealth teams, both clinical and technical, with a systematic approach and common language to proactively recognize their strengths, weaknesses, and gaps in service development, implementation, and management.

This guide will introduce the phases and key concepts of TSIM and provide foundational knowledge on how to establish the organizational structure and governance to successfully develop and manage telehealth services. Simultaneously, a fictional provider organization, *Ohio River Health System*, will be followed to demonstrate the TSIM concepts in action while developing and implementing telehealth services (see Appendix). Telehealth holds the potential to significantly improve the way healthcare is delivered and accessed, and TSIM provides the roadmap for national digital transformation that results in telehealth for efficient, effective, and higher-quality care for patients.

1.2 Brief history of telehealth

The modern-day version of telehealth originated as early as 1948 with the short-distance transmission of radiologic images by telephone lines between West Chester and Philadelphia, Pennsylvania. Medical video communications began in 1959 when clinicians at the University of Nebraska used two-way interactive television to send neurological examinations across campus. In 1963, Massachusetts General Hospital established a telecommunications link to connect its providers with a medical station staffed by nurses at Logan Airport.

As many of these programs continued to mature throughout the 1960s and 1970s, the US government, with an interest in delivering medical services to astronauts and rural, isolated areas, began to invest significant funding into telehealth research through the Department of Health, Education and Welfare (now known as the Department of Health and Human Services, or DHHS) and the National Aeronautics and Space Administration (NASA).

Unfortunately, a majority of the early investments made, and programs started, were not sustainable, and interest in telehealth appeared to decline in the 1980s. In the 1990s, enthusiasm in telehealth began to reemerge with the increased adoption of the internet. National organizations and federal departments devoted to telehealth began to organize, and teleradiology and telepsychiatry began to achieve broad adoption. Teleradiology has been so successful that it has become a standard of radiology care and is rarely even referred to as "telehealth" anymore.[6,7]

In the 2000s, state and federal agencies continued to push for and invest in technological advancements in healthcare. Specifically, significant federal investments were made to catalyze the adoption of electronic health records. In addition, federal funding was allocated to establish telehealth resource centers across the US to help navigate the complexities of telehealth adoption. While some states began to organize their own telehealth networks, the delivery of telehealth was still limited to innovators in the field.

The Affordable Care Act (ACA) was enacted in 2010,[8] initiating a transformational movement towards a value-based healthcare system. While the transition away from the historical fee-for-service (FFS) reimbursement system continued at a slow pace, the ACA inspired a new wave of early telehealth adopters as forward-thinking health systems began to invest their own resources in telehealth infrastructure and services.

1.3   The pandemic shift to virtual

In 2020, healthcare organizations across the world experienced a historic explosion of telehealth utilization, fueled by the COVID-19 pandemic and telehealth waivers in the US that removed many historical regulatory barriers. The pendulum of healthcare encounters swung heavily into virtual care out of a necessity to minimize further risk of exposure to the virus. Healthcare organizations across the US demonstrated significant increases in telehealth utilization.[9] At the federal level, the Centers for Medicare and Medicaid Services (CMS) published a report that noted that 43.5% of Medicare primary care visits in April 2020 were conducted via telehealth, compared with only 0.1% in February 2020.[10] The pandemic helped advance telehealth years along the adoption curve. Many patients and providers were using telehealth for the very first time, opening their eyes to its potential for patient convenience and provider efficiency. According to a McKinsey report, about 20% of healthcare could be conducted virtually.[11]

But as the pandemic evolved and clinics started to reopen, the pendulum began to shift back towards in-person care. It was clear that a hybrid model (i.e. a combination of telehealth and in-person healthcare) was going to be part of the new normal. However, the shift back to in-person care exposed many of the vulnerabilities in the rapid telehealth implementations that occurred over the previous year.

Early in the pandemic, many organizations distributed a simple workflow and a video client to their physicians in the rush of the emergency. Other organizations encouraged providers to move to telephone interactions exclusively. In fact, about one-third of the Medicare beneficiaries who received a telehealth visit only received a telephone call.[12] In addition, providers were concerned about how they would navigate the end of the public health emergency waivers that removed many of the regulatory and payment barriers.[13] Unless there was an existing telehealth infrastructure already established, most organizations did not have the time to methodically develop and implement their telehealth services, and most of the emergent telehealth capabilities were developed external to, and not integrated with, their traditional delivery system.

1.4 Historical challenges to telehealth development and implementation

Unfortunately, many of the challenges that impaired the success of telehealth pioneers were never fully overcome. The technical, behavioral, economic, and organizational barriers identified in the late 1990s persist more than 20 years later.[14,15] While a foundation of principles was established for successfully developing telehealth systems, most organizations lacked a standard approach to implement those principles into action consistently. Common themes that influence successful integration of telehealth services have been identified. However, without a common guiding approach and nomenclature, healthcare organizations continue to struggle with successfully developing and implementing telehealth services.[16]

While the COVID-19 pandemic catalyzed an unprecedented level of telehealth adoption out of necessity, the majority of the rapid implementations were temporary solutions and not a standardized approach in developing high-quality, sustainable services integrated into the traditional delivery system. The pandemic also highlighted existing health disparities involving digital technology, health literacy, and internet access that should be accounted for and addressed in new telehealth delivery models.[17] While the pendulum of telehealth utilization initially swung high during major shifts towards virtual care, organizations then began to experience the pullback and struggled to navigate how to establish a hybrid in-person and telehealth model.[18,19] As investments in telehealth technologies continue to hit all-time record highs, it is advantageous for healthcare organizations to invest in the education and training of personnel who will be charged with developing and implementing the successful telehealth services[20] that will transform clinical care delivery.

1.5 History of the MUSC Center for Telehealth and the creation of TSIM

The MUSC began its telehealth journey in 2005 with an innovative endeavor to improve maternal fetal health in a rural, medically underserved region of the state.[21] Shortly thereafter, a telestroke network began development in an area of the US known as the Stroke Belt. Over an eight-year period, physician innovators at MUSC continued to develop telehealth services through grassroots initiatives and ad-hoc funding mechanisms to mitigate health disparities across South Carolina. In 2013, with around a dozen MUSC telehealth services functioning at different levels of maturity, the South Carolina Legislature invested telehealth funding through MUSC. MUSC was charged with creating a statewide telehealth network and developing telehealth services that addressed the needs of South Carolina communities.

Catalyzed by the state support, the MUSC Center for Telehealth (the "Center") was founded in 2013, and an effort to organize the existing telehealth services was initiated. Simultaneously, the Center led an organizational movement to rapidly develop telehealth services across the health system. In addition to the state's legislative mandate, MUSC's chief executive officer asserted a bold vision that "any clinical services we deliver *inside* our walls, we should be able to deliver *outside* our walls."

In a parallel effort, the Center organized a statewide strategic planning process to engage telehealth stakeholders from across the state. In 2014, MUSC published the first statewide telehealth strategic plan, resulting in the creation of the South Carolina Telehealth Alliance (SCTA). The SCTA, headquartered at MUSC, is a statewide collaborative bonded by a shared vison that *telehealth will grow to support the delivery of healthcare to all South Carolinians*. The SCTA was later recognized by the American Telemedicine Association as the sole winner of its 2019 President's Award for Transformation of Healthcare Delivery.[22]

As MUSC pushed for rapid adoption of telehealth services across the organization, the Center began to experience growing pains due to structural and process deficiencies. Shawn Valenta, who became MUSC's first Director of Telehealth in 2013, had previously demonstrated nationally recognized success in structure and process improvements when leading initiatives within MUSC's respiratory therapy (RT) department.[23] Valenta led a high-performing RT team through initiatives that resulted in MUSC being one of only three respiratory care departments in the US recognized by the University Health Consortium (UHC, now known as Vizient) for significant cost reduction and quality improvement.

As a former advanced cardiovascular life support instructor, Valenta was used to working in collaborative teams using common terminology, algorithms, and protocols to efficiently manage complex medical emergencies, but equivalent standards for developing and implementing telehealth services seemed absent in the industry. Valenta began to research telehealth development and implementation models, but found limited information beyond what MUSC's experience had already revealed. The article "A review of telehealth service implementation frameworks" by Liezl Van Dyk further validated the lack of a comprehensive, practical roadmap for telehealth service implementation, and Valenta agreed with Van Dyk's conclusion that "a holistic implementation approach" was needed.[24] Concurrently, MUSC had begun an information technology (IT) service management initiative adopting the ITIL® framework and Valenta had seen the benefits of using a shared language and common set of principles and practices.[25] The convergence of these factors helped Valenta and other MUSC leaders recognize that the best way to help the Center develop and implement sustainable telehealth services was to create its own holistic telehealth framework based on their standardized processes and common terminology.

With the support of a standardized approach to telehealth service development, MUSC grew telehealth interactions to nationally recognized volumes and demonstrated substantial improvements in patient outcomes. It also rapidly expanded existing services and concurrently developed new telehealth programs. It became known for both breadth and depth of telehealth services, and in 2017 received the distinction of being one of the first National Telehealth Centers of Excellence in the US.[26] This federal designation, offered by the HRSA, also came with funding to invest in the continued development and rigorous scientific evaluation of telehealth services. Through these efforts and the journey of continuous quality improvement, MUSC has matured the TSIM framework such that it can inform the telehealth aspirations of any health system or provider.

1.6 Purpose of the TSIM guide

This TSIM guide is intended for telehealth leaders and teams that are responsible for their organization's digital transformation efforts. These efforts could be large-scale, full-enterprise adoption of telehealth services, or simply improving on the direct-to-patient ambulatory telehealth services that were implemented during the pandemic. Either way, telehealth teams must navigate the complexities of telehealth service development and implementation that transect almost every department in the organization.

TSIM serves as a roadmap to successfully develop, implement, and sustain telehealth services. It provides an architecture and terminology to boost the clinical and technical collaboration required to successfully design high-quality, highly reliable telehealth services that are integrated into the traditional care delivery system. In addition, it provides strategic principles and philosophies that aid in redesigning care delivery and not simply using video to replicate the existing inefficiencies of in-person processes. Finally, it helps teams identify strengths and weaknesses within their structure and processes for continued improvement. With significant investments being made in telehealth technologies, TSIM is an investment into the people who are charged with deploying and integrating these technologies into user-friendly and financially sustainable models of care delivery.

2 | Technology

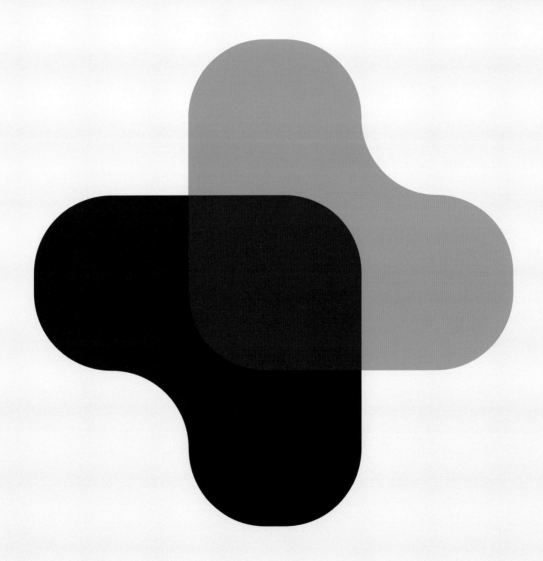

2.1 Telehealth modes of care delivery

Telehealth modes of delivery are often categorized in diverse ways with two main themes: synchronous and asynchronous communication technology. These themes can then be subdivided into subcategories: real-time encounters, remote patient monitoring, store and forward, and mobile health (see Figure 2.1). While the traditional synchronous (i.e. real-time encounters) and asynchronous (i.e. store and forward) telehealth technology models are focused on a single healthcare interaction over distance, remote patient monitoring (RPM) and mobile health (mHealth) applications are focused on the management of health over a continuum of time.

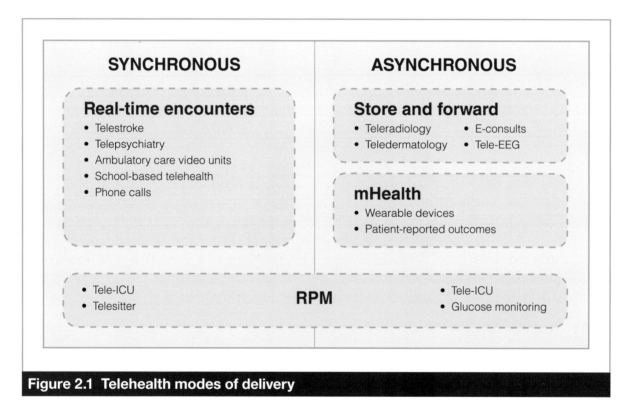

Figure 2.1 Telehealth modes of delivery

2.1.1 Synchronous "real-time" encounters

Synchronous technologies, or those that facilitate a real-time exchange, use audio-only (i.e. telephone) or two-way audio-video functionality. Synchronous encounters are the traditional delivery of what most people envision when discussing telehealth. Telestroke and telepsychiatry are examples of synchronous encounters to treat individual patients in real time. Additional peripheral devices and information-gathering systems can add to evaluation capabilities and otherwise support the synchronous interaction. Strategic considerations that drive the use of synchronous technologies include visual (video) connections to establish rapport, billing compliance regulations, clinical assessment needs, and, in some states, the legal benefit of establishing physician-patient relationships.

2.1.2 Asynchronous – store and forward

Asynchronous store-and-forward technologies allow communication and data exchange that occurs as a transmission in which the content is viewable at a later time. These technologies may leverage a one-way transmission or two-way exchanges. Common uses include remote interpretations of locally performed procedures (e.g. tele-EEG), collaboration and consultation from provider to provider (e.g. e-consults), and the transmission of images and information that support longitudinal care decisions (e.g. telewound care). One of the drivers of considering asynchronous approaches is a need for higher efficiencies in the use of provider capacity and in clinical workflows that are primarily dependent on the transmission of discrete and well-defined information. Asynchronous technologies may also provide added efficiencies to the use of the workforce, and can often offer benefits of added convenience and ease of use relative to synchronous processes.

2.1.3 Remote patient monitoring

Remote patient monitoring is a mode of telehealth in which a discrete set of patient data such as symptoms, vital signs, or other physiologic measures is transmitted and organized to be reviewed by a monitoring healthcare team, in order to apply subsequent care plan changes to optimize the patient's health. This technological approach can be delivered in an outpatient setting (e.g. home glucose monitoring for diabetic patients) using asynchronous technologies, or in an inpatient setting with real-time, synchronous video monitoring (e.g. telesitter). Tele-ICU is an example of an RPM service that uses both synchronous (e.g. real-time video monitoring) and asynchronous (e.g. sending images and lab data) technologies to provide a comprehensive telehealth service. Remote monitoring approaches are often considered when the focused management of one or more health conditions in a population is of primary importance. Increasingly, as reimbursement innovations progress, remote monitoring in the outpatient setting is being applied to augment encounter-based care in between visits.

2.1.4 Mobile health

The final telehealth technology category, an asynchronous solution, is mobile health (or mHealth), in which information from a patient is generated via an application on a mobile device, such as a smartphone with internet connectivity. Mobile health is opening up new diagnostic capabilities through wearable technology and patient-reported outcomes (PROs). Wearable technology devices (e.g. a smart watch) can collect, analyze, and transmit patient health data (e.g. heart rate, mobility). PROs provide the ability to gather a patient's subjective assessment of their health status via questionnaires (e.g. symptom tracking). In addition, mHealth can make information available through secure messaging to assess the health and well-being of a patient. Strategic implications to the use of these approaches include population health interventions such as the monitoring of viral symptoms across a community, and the management of health conditions in individuals in which deteriorations in personal functioning, such as neurological conditions, can prompt interventions.

2.2 Telehealth technology solutions

Telehealth technology solutions fall within three main categories: telehealth software, video endpoints, and peripheral devices. The telehealth software is what is used to conduct online communication between patient and provider, or from provider to provider. It can be as simple as a two-way audio-video connection, or it can also offer additional functionality such as online scheduling, virtual waiting rooms, documentation, and payment capabilities. Video endpoints are the hardware devices that are used at both the patient and provider locations and where the two-way audio-video connection occurs. Examples of video endpoints include telehealth carts, laptops, tablets, and smartphones. Peripheral devices are telehealth medical devices that are used to assist the visit with capturing additional clinical information like heart or lung sounds.

2.2.1 Telehealth software

Telehealth software solutions may provide a broad range of functionality and have historically been targeted at supporting specific use cases. Telehealth software that supports a telestroke encounter may include a real-time two-way audio-video connection, dual documentation, and image exchange capabilities (e.g. sending CT scans through the platform). Dual documentation is when both originating site and distant site providers can document in a single note within the platform. Other telehealth solutions are tailored more towards patient-initiated, "direct-to-consumer" encounters. Direct-to-consumer platforms may include both synchronous (e.g. video, phone) and asynchronous (e.g. patient intake, chat) functionalities.

While it is theoretically optimal to have one telehealth software solution that meets all needs, organizations are likely to encounter challenges in finding a technology platform with all the capabilities they require. Many telehealth vendors may claim to be an enterprise solution, but telehealth services have different requirements depending on where the patient is located and the supporting functionality needed. While there is an active acquisition race to achieve the enterprise solution vision, the reality is that some telehealth platforms are stronger in certain areas than others. Ideally, the technology should enable the process rather than dictate it.

In order to navigate this current state, an "intentional fragmentation" approach can be applied in which the best technologies for each use case are selected to support the respective clinical strategies. This may mean that one telehealth platform is selected for hospital services and another for direct-to-consumer telehealth services. Intentional fragmentation is intended to be a short-term strategy as telehealth solutions are matured to meet all clinical delivery needs. Organizations applying this approach should outline a long-term technology roadmap to achieve eventual consolidation and interoperability.

2.2.2 Video endpoints

A video endpoint is the physical hardware device at each end of a video conferencing system. In telehealth, physical endpoints are at the patient originating site and the distant site where the provider is located. Examples of video endpoints may include smartphones, tablets, laptops, desktop computers, and telehealth carts. Some telehealth software solutions will not work on certain video endpoints. Also, the video endpoint's camera may have additional functionality such as pan-tilt-zoom or far-end camera control that allows the clinical providers at the distant site to better assess the patient. When determining the technical requirements, it is important that the clinical providers understand the video endpoint's capabilities to ensure the device meets the clinical needs for a successful visit.

2.2.3 Peripheral devices

Peripheral devices ("peripherals") are telehealth medical devices used to gather additional clinical information (e.g. heart rate, blood pressure, lung/heart sounds) during the telehealth encounter to assist with the diagnosis. They can be used in conjunction with real-time video or to support RPM models, and can assist with clinical decision-making. Examples of peripheral devices include digital examination cameras, Bluetooth stethoscopes and otoscopes, electronic weight scales, digital pulse oximetry, and electronic blood pressure cuffs.

2.3 Technology selection process

Many healthcare organizations start their telehealth journey with procuring a telehealth platform. Leading with a technology is a cardinal sin in telehealth. A core principle in TSIM is to "think technology last." This means that the strategy and clinical needs of the service drive the technology solution requirements, not the other way around. Too often, technology enthusiasts fall into the trap of "shiny toy syndrome" and become blinded, and eventually led, by the technical capabilities of a telehealth platform or device. The selection of telehealth technologies should always originate from the clinical, operational, and technical needs required to achieve the telehealth strategy (see Figure 2.2). Given the investment of resources required to obtain and install telehealth technologies, a formal request for information (RFI) or request for proposal (RFP) process can be conducted to procure telehealth technologies. The RFI or RFP process provides an invitation to the telehealth technology industry and allows for an objective, inclusive scan for the telehealth solution that will best meet the needs of the organization and its clinical telehealth strategy.

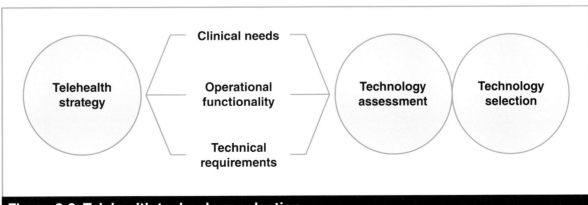

Figure 2.2 Telehealth technology selection

The RFI or RFP document provides an overview of the organization and telehealth department, clearly articulates the telehealth goals and scope of services to be delivered, identifies the technology requirements, and provides instructions on the overall process. To eliminate vendors that do not meet the minimum requirements, a screening process is conducted. Vendor finalists then conduct demonstrations of their solutions for a small group of telehealth stakeholders representing different perspectives (e.g. clinical, operational, technical). The telehealth stakeholder team objectively scores the vendor finalists on predetermined criteria (see Table 2.1). Considering that some criteria are more important than others, it is common to use a weighted scoring system and place a heavier (i.e. higher value) weight on the elements with the highest priority.

Table 2.1 Example scoring criteria for a telehealth solution RFI/RFP process

Category	Category topics
Vendor qualifications	Company background and history Company's experience in the industry Company's customer base and reference list Company's technology development roadmap
Product qualifications	Product capabilities Integration opportunities Information security and regulatory compliance Data reporting Patient and provider experience and workflow
Demonstrated success	Client experience Utilization and scalability Training and implementation plan
Overall cost of the solution	Upfront/implementation costs Recurring costs Upgrade/maintenance costs

2.4 Connectivity

Stable internet connectivity is vital to achieving a successful telehealth encounter. When telehealth services with real-time video capabilities are being delivered into rural locations or into a patient's home, connectivity issues may arise if there is inadequate broadband access. "Broadband" refers to a high-speed internet connection. According to the Federal Communications Commission (FCC), it is defined as internet connectivity with at least 25 Mbps (megabits per second) download speed and at least 3 Mbps upload speed. In addition to broadband, adequate bandwidth is essential, especially when conducting a real-time synchronous video encounter. Network bandwidth is the amount of data that can be transmitted across a network's path in a given time period. As more healthcare (and services in other industries) moves online, the competition for bandwidth access gets challenging. Asynchronous technologies typically do not require as much broadband or bandwidth as synchronous technologies, and that flexibility may impact technology decisions in the Strategy phase. Conducting a network connectivity assessment with new partners or into new regions will highlight technical challenges and aid in selecting the right technology to implement for a given telehealth service.[27]

2.5 Information security

In order to successfully scale telehealth services, patients must trust that their interactions with their providers and the transmissions of their health information will be secure.[28] If not protected appropriately, telehealth services can be a significant cybersecurity risk for patients and health systems. The basic principles of information security include confidentiality, integrity, and availability.[29] When selecting a telehealth platform, it is imperative to ensure that the technology is compliant with the Health Insurance Portability and Accountability Act (HIPAA) and keeps the data confidential. In addition, deploying the telehealth services on a secure network that is continuously monitored for risks helps keep the data accurate, maintaining data integrity. Finally, availability focuses on ensuring that authorized users have access to the platform and data. Implementing an identity authentication process (e.g. two-factor authentication) to access the platform can provide an extra layer of security. Overall, it is imperative to partner with information security personnel to establish a security policy that governs all telehealth technologies and services deployed.

2.6 Interoperability

When selecting a telehealth platform, it is important to understand its interoperability capabilities (i.e. its ability to electronically share and receive data from other health information systems). One example of interoperability is implementing single sign-on (SSO), in which users within an organization can maintain a single login name and password for multiple trusted applications. This can help with the user-friendliness of a new telehealth platform. In addition, integration with the health system's electronic health record (EHR) to enable pushing and pulling of health information can substantially improve the quality of the clinical encounter.

The pushing and pulling of health information occurs through an application programming interface (API). An API is a set of standards that dictate how software applications can communicate and exchange information.[30] APIs to connect telehealth platforms and EHRs have historically used an HL7 (Health Level 7) interface, but more recently, telehealth platforms that can use Fast Healthcare Interoperability Resources (FHIR, pronounced as "fire") to integrate to electronic health records provide a promising and more efficient opportunity to securely exchange discrete healthcare data. As interoperability continues to evolve, the coordination of healthcare delivery will mature with it.

3 | People

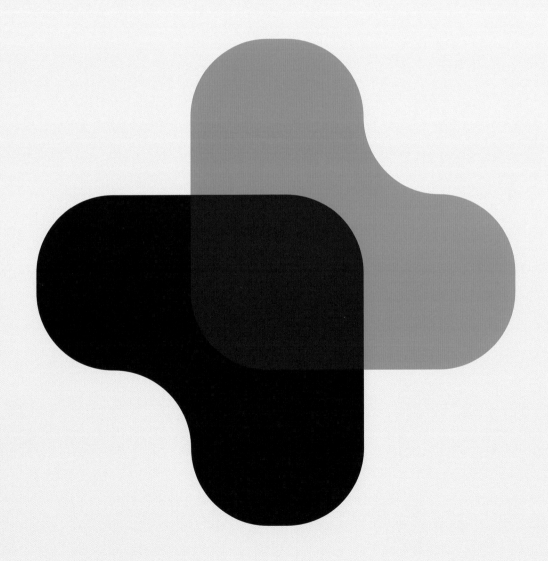

3.1 Building organizational structure and governance

In order to successfully support clinical transformation efforts using TSIM, it is vital to create an organizational structure with effective governance that is integrated and aligned with the overall health system. Too often, telehealth departments are established as teams siloed from the organization, with their own strategic plan and goals that may or may not align with the overall system's priorities. Similarly, many organizations treat telehealth implementations like an IT project, with limited clinical expertise involvement. Telehealth technology solutions cannot parachute into existing clinical practice with expectations of sustained success. Effective telehealth services are led by clinical champions and administrative leaders who understand the current delivery of healthcare and can account for the many complex factors (c.g. technology, legal, reimbursement) that can impact the success of a telehealth service.

A centralized telehealth governance model can maintain a structure of decision points, process ownership, and transparent accountability of departmental and service development decision-making. While establishing governance through a system of committees may differ by organization, some examples of core telehealth processes that often benefit from structured decision-making are technology strategy, business sustainability, compliance, change management, and service quality. An inclusive forum for open communication and collaboration between telehealth team members will expedite informed decision-making.

3.2 Clinical champions

Telehealth services need clinical champions who understand the current clinical workflow, can articulate the goals of care, and can help navigate the challenges of implementation and change management. Telehealth technology solutions provide a new tool for clinicians to reach and treat their patients in a more efficient and effective way, but they must be collaboratively developed, effectively implemented, and continuously improved to achieve full potential. Identifying clinical champions with optimism and willingness to innovate is essential. The positive attitude of a process-oriented clinical champion is infectious, and helps the teams work through the inevitable early workflow and system optimizations required for a service to run efficiently. If the clinical champion becomes overly discouraged by the telehealth process and the support received, the broader clinical team will soon follow, and service engagement will be difficult to recover. The power and influence of clinical champion engagement and leadership consistently proves to be one of the most impactful factors to early and long-term service success, thus warranting substantial investment in time and resources.

3.3 Telehealth administrative leader

The TSIM guide is aimed at supporting telehealth administrative leaders and the teams they manage. The administrative leader is charged with supporting their clinical champions in making an initial telehealth idea turn into a successful, sustainable telehealth service. Administrative leaders must navigate their teams through the matrix of stakeholders that are required to successfully develop, implement, and sustain telehealth services. In addition to clinical and IT expertise, administrative leaders benefit from having foundational knowledge in strategic planning, project management, education and training, clinical operations, revenue cycle, billing compliance, health law, procurement, government relations, data analytics, business analysis, and process improvement. While the administrative leader may not have personal expertise in these many areas, they should know the local resources and experts who can address each of these topics.

3.4 Telehealth team formation

A holistic approach, leveraging dedicated resources and collaborating expertise, is essential to successfully create and manage telehealth services. Decisions on which roles are created centrally versus collaboratively allocated to telehealth should be made locally and dependent on the breadth and depth of the planned and operational telehealth services.

A centralized team, established to support the development, implementation, and ongoing support of the organization's telehealth services, provides for a strong foundation to support clinical transformation efforts. While the size and scope of a telehealth department will vary depending on the organization's range of services and strategic imperatives, the goal is to manage resources more effectively through structure and coordination.

Many telehealth departments have been started as a "department of one," meaning one person was charged with being the organizational expert in telehealth to help advance their institution's goals. That role can mature in different ways, depending on the person, presence of clinical champions, organizational support, and available resources. As the telehealth department begins to grow with new services and team members, responsibilities begin to divide into specific areas of expertise. While many healthcare organizations have different approaches on which duties should be centralized within the telehealth team, there are certain responsibilities in which dedicated telehealth personnel can be advantageous for standardized development, implementation, and operations. Concurrently, there are roles and functions best obtained through collaboration between the telehealth team and other organizational departments (see Table 3.1).

Table 3.1 Telehealth team formation

Responsibilities central to core telehealth team	Skillsets to absorb into core team with growth	Expertise best obtained through collaboration
Telehealth service development	Business analysis	Legal
Training	Marketing	Compliance
Education	Data analytics	Government relations
Business management	Technical support*	Payor relations
Telehealth technology – systems/software	Telehealth network Infrastructure	Electronic health record
Partner outreach	Business development	Medical staff affairs
Telehealth service management	Outcomes reporting	Information security

* Telehealth technical support can be outsourced through vendor or third-party contractual relationships.

3.5 Communication and collaboration

As successful telehealth delivery is often fueled by effective collaboration, formalizing the principles of business relationship management can aid in maintaining positive relationships with both internal and external stakeholders. Internal stakeholders may include the consultant providers (e.g. physicians, advanced practice providers) and interorganizational personnel from complementary departments (e.g. legal, procurement) that may impact the successful development and implementation of telehealth services. External stakeholders include customers of the telehealth service (e.g. patients, external providers) and other related parties (e.g. partnering hospitals, third-party payors, state medical board) that may impact the success of the service.

Outreach and engagement with stakeholders will strengthen a telehealth team's ability to navigate some of the complex challenges of service development and implementation. For example, a clinical champion conducting provider-to-provider conversations can make a positive impact with the initial implementation of the service. The clinical champion can use initial meetings and training activities to assist with buy-in, establish collegial relationships, and answer any questions about the new telehealth service. Telehealth can significantly improve the delivery of high-quality care and increase access for underserved populations, but these results are difficult to achieve without building trust and successful partnerships with community providers.

3.6 Responsibility chart

Since telehealth development and implementation can be very challenging in navigating different stakeholders, TSIM recommends using a responsibility chart to clearly define who is responsible (R), accountable (A), consulted (C), and informed (I) at each step throughout the process. The responsibility chart will help communicate roles and responsibilities and ensure key stakeholders are consulted and informed at vital steps along the way. In the example in Table 3.2, the role of a project manager is the accountable owner for all of the steps identified. The responsibility chart clearly identifies who will be responsible for completing each task, and they are also responsible for consulting with and informing other key stakeholders.

Table 3.2 Example of a responsibility chart

	Clinical champion	Project manager	Clinical informaticist	Business manager	Training coordinator
Contract	C	A	C	R	I
Clinical workflow	C	A	R	C	C
Technology system changes	C	A	R	C	I
Scheduling protocols	C	A	R	I	I
Training plan	C	A	C	I	R

R = Responsible; A = Accountable; C = Consulted; I = Informed

4 | Legal and regulatory

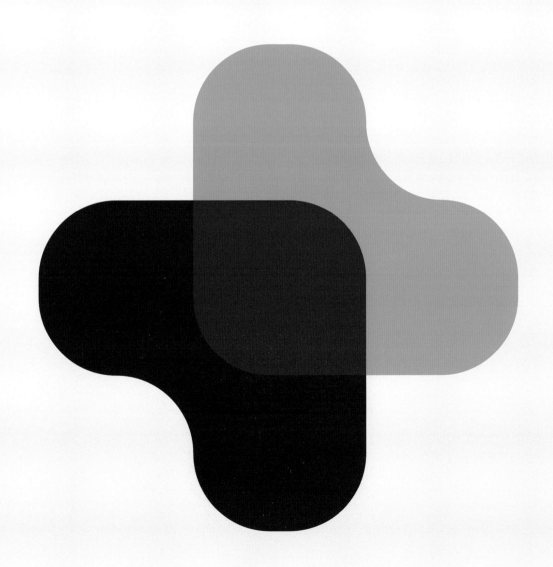

When developing telehealth services, both state and federal laws and regulations must be understood and considered. This chapter covers foundational legal and regulatory terms and definitions that inform the telehealth service development process. Administrative telehealth leaders must be knowledgeable of these legal concepts prior to initiating services through the TSIM framework, and know when to seek counsel from legal and compliance experts.

4.1 Medical licensure

In the US, clinical providers must be licensed in both the state where they physically practice medicine and the state where the patient is located (i.e. the "originating site") in order to deliver telehealth services to that patient. While there are some exceptions to this rule, as each state has its own laws (e.g. bordering state reciprocity, follow-up care allowances), having a medical license in the state where the patient is located is a core requirement to deliver telehealth services if there is no exception. Furthermore, each state has its own medical board and unique licensure requirements. Thus, if the strategy is to develop a telehealth service with multi-state reach, it is important to invest in robust medical staff support to optimize the efficiency of multi-state licensure.

4.2 Malpractice insurance coverage

To mitigate potential liability risks, it is important to review the malpractice insurance coverage for the consulting providers delivering the telehealth services to ensure that the current coverage includes the telehealth services intended to be delivered. In addition, if the telehealth service is intended to be delivered in a different state than where the provider traditionally delivers care, they may need additional or extended malpractice insurance coverage to safeguard against potentially higher liability risks.

4.3 Credentialing and privileging

If telehealth services are to be delivered in a hospital, the clinical providers must be credentialed and privileged to deliver that care. This includes completing and submitting credentialing information to the hospital's medical staff office, which will review the information and verify that the providers meet the necessary qualifications.

In addition to credentialing, the provider must also be privileged to practice in their area of specialty. The process of privileging documents the provider's competency in their area of care. If a telehealth service is planned to be scaled to multiple hospitals, credentialing and privileging can be extremely resource-intensive, duplicative, and costly. In 2011, the Joint Commission and the Centers for Medicare & Medicaid Services (CMS) approved a "credentialing-by-proxy" process that allows for the originating site hospital to accept the consulting provider's hospital credentialing and privileging process. This process has been an effective tool for telehealth providers partnering with different hospital systems.[31]

4.4 Standard of care

The standard of care is defined legally as a degree of care that a reasonable person should exercise under similar circumstances.[32] While the standard of care in medicine continues to evolve and is sensitive to people, places, and time, the standard of care in telehealth is consistent with the standard of care delivered in person.[33] If a physical assessment is required for a diagnosis, a diagnosis should not be completed without that assessment. In telehealth delivery models, the traditional physical examination could be performed by licensed onsite providers or by using peripheral devices. If a provider cannot make a clear examination via telehealth, an in-person visit should be scheduled.

4.5 Patient-provider relationship

A clinical provider establishes a patient-provider relationship once the provider serves a patient's medical needs.[34] It is important to understand the local state laws on establishing a patient-provider relationship via telehealth. Many states allow a patient-provider relationship to be established via telehealth,[35] but they may come with additional guidance, such as medical prescribing restrictions on relationships that are established solely via telehealth.

4.6 Prescribing medications via telehealth

All states allow providers to prescribe medications via telehealth as long as the provider complies with the state's local rules on establishing a patient-provider relationship. However, it is important to understand the local and federal rules, as certain restrictions may apply (e.g. prescribing controlled substances). For example, the Ryan Haight Act, intended to combat rogue internet prescribing practices, has historically placed federal restrictions on prescribing controlled substances via online interactions.[36] Unintentionally, the Act has impeded some use cases of clinically appropriate care from being delivered via telehealth, by requiring an initial in-person visit. Recently, there has been some federal movement to allow prescribing of controlled substances via telehealth in an effort to assist with the treatment of opioid addiction.

4.7 Informed consent

In addition to the basic medical consent for treatment, there are evolving regulations on obtaining an informed consent, either written or verbal, from patients receiving telehealth services. Reasons for the consent include informing the patient that they can refuse the telehealth services and request an in-person visit, or that they may be required to pay an additional co-pay for the services. It is important to learn the state and federal laws, along with any third-party payor requirements with regard to obtaining patient consent for telehealth services.

4.8 Documentation and medical records

Telehealth providers are expected to meet the same requirements for medical record documentation and record-keeping as they would for in-person encounters. When a collaborating provider from a different organization is treating a patient via telehealth within a healthcare setting, documentation of the telehealth encounter must be maintained within the patient originating site's EHR (i.e. the legal medical record). How the providers will document for the telehealth service should be carefully considered, with plans developed for how clinical documentation of the telehealth encounter will be incorporated into the legal medical record.

When the telehealth provider does not share a common EHR with the patient originating site, this issue can become quite complex. There are two common approaches to addressing this issue. One option is to have the consulting provider trained to document directly in the originating site's EHR. If there are multiple originating sites with different EHRs, provider satisfaction and engagement will suffer, and it will be challenging to scale the service. Second, numerous telehealth technologies provide documentation tools in their platforms. When the documentation occurs in a third-party telehealth software product, the telehealth provider's documentation note can be sent to the originating site's EHR, either automatically through an API integration or through a manual process. While it is not legally required to keep a copy of the telehealth encounter at the consulting provider's organization (i.e. the distant site), the benefits of maintaining these records include an institution's own record-keeping as proactive protection against any future malpractice claims, and to preserve additional patient history context if the patient is ever transferred to the telehealth provider's hospital in the future.

4.9 Stark Law and Anti-Kickback Statute

Laws to consider when drafting a telehealth agreement include the Stark Law, Anti-Kickback Statute, and any applicable state and federal regulations.[37] The Stark Law was instituted with the passing of the Ethics in Patient Referrals Acts of 1989, and was intended to prevent physicians from referring Medicare beneficiaries to entities in which they, or an immediate family member, have a financial relationship. The Anti-Kickback Statute makes it illegal to provide or receive payments for inducing referrals for healthcare services reimbursable by Medicare or Medicaid. Historically, providing free telehealth equipment to partnering sites or patients has been scrutinized by the Health and Human Services' Office of the Inspector General (OIG), but new safe harbors have been approved that permit some in-kind remuneration to support care coordination. While these exceptions and safe harbor laws exist, it is recommended that legal counsel reviews all arrangements to mitigate any unintended legal risk.

4.10 Fair market value

Telehealth transactions and agreements must be consistent with fair market value (FMV) pricing. It is beneficial for organizations to document their methodology in establishing FMV pricing for their telehealth services. It is also recommended to regularly conduct an FMV analysis for the telehealth services being delivered and for any financial transactions to support the services (e.g. internal physician compensation). As telehealth adoption increases, the overall cost of the services delivered may be impacted, and a regularly scheduled FMV determination will help ensure that the financial transactions and agreements are still compliant with applicable laws.

4.11 Patient confidentiality and HIPAA

While telehealth offers the promise of improving healthcare through more efficient and effective delivery of care, patient privacy and information security risks must be accounted for and addressed, not only to meet state and federal regulations but also to ensure patient and provider trust is maintained.[38] When the physical endpoint on the patient's side is their own mobile device (e.g. a smartphone), the risk is elevated as the device is outside the control of a preferred closed information security environment.

Information security personnel assess and mitigate risks to maintain compliance with protecting patient health information (PHI). As with any healthcare service, compliance with the HIPAA Privacy Rule[39] is federally required. Only authorized users should have access to PHI. Secure telehealth connections are implemented and monitored to protect against breaches. When a health system is using a telehealth platform from a third-party vendor, they are required to execute a Business Associate Agreement with that vendor to outline data storage and security protections and compliance with all HIPAA regulations.

5 | Sustainability

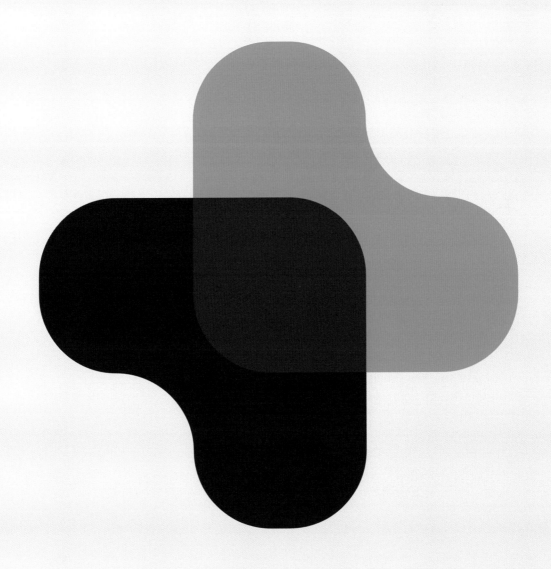

Telehealth services have had a long history of sustainability challenges due to limited reimbursement policies and poor business planning. TSIM establishes sustainability planning in the Strategy phase. As reimbursement is often cited as one of the top challenges of telehealth adoption, creating sustainable business models in a shifting healthcare payment system can be challenging. This chapter covers telehealth business models that support service sustainability.

5.1 Financial management

Financial management is the function that fulfills the financial administrative duties so that the telehealth department can successfully achieve its objectives. Financial management functions may include planning, budgeting, forecasting, reporting, establishing service pricing and business models, return on investment (ROI) and value on investment (VOI) analysis, accounts payable, and accounts receivable. Through effective financial management, successful business models to fund the operations and growth of the telehealth services may be supported by direct revenues, indirect revenues, alternative payment models, or funding from alternative sources.

5.2 Direct revenues

Direct revenues may include payments from third-party payors, contractual payments from partnering organizations receiving telehealth services, or self-pay from the patients. Direct revenue from third-party payors, including both government and commercial payors, typically comes in the form of an encounter-based code under the traditional fee-for-service system. Contractual revenues may come from a partner hospital that is paying an on-call and/or "per encounter" fee to a telehealth provider organization that is delivering a service that may otherwise not be attainable at that location. Cash payments from patients, often referred to as "out of pocket," are seen in many direct-to-consumer telehealth models, specifically virtual urgent care, where patients have been willing to pay for the convenience.

5.3 Indirect revenues

Indirect revenue streams to consider include benefit to the institutional enterprise from additional patient engagement and broadening of the reach of the clinical services offered. Telehealth initiatives may also improve the quality and process metrics that can enable larger returns for shared risk payments. Cost reduction strategies are also common for telehealth services. Added efficiencies in care delivery may decrease costs in bundled payment opportunities. Strategies to reduce hospital readmissions, or other penalties, are also common areas of focus for telehealth. Aligning the benefits from one arm of the health system to telehealth intervention can lead to support for a telehealth program that may otherwise be seen as a cost burden.

5.4 Alternative payment models

As the payment for care continues to transition away from the historical fee-for-service reimbursement system, the use of telehealth is increasing in newly developed alternative payment models.[40] The two most common of these are accountable care organizations (ACOs) and bundled payments. An ACO model establishes an agreement between a healthcare organization and a third-party payor in which the payments for care are connected to patient outcomes. Bundling involves packaging multiple services across the care continuum into one single payment (e.g. for knee surgery). Both models help advance progress towards more value-based care, and telehealth is a strategic care delivery tool being deployed at healthcare organizations adopting these alternative payment models.

5.5 Value on investment

The creation of a value case for any healthcare service can be a complex process, and often, telehealth services may not clearly demonstrate a traditional return on investment, especially in an FFS reimbursement model that may not fully reward preventative services. When the value proposition of a telehealth service is diverse and challenging to interpret, a value-on-investment equation can be used to define a quantifiable and easy-to-interpret target that all stakeholders can agree on.[41] At the simplest level, the telehealth VOI is equal to the impact of the service divided by the cost invested. The primary impact of the service may be an increase in access to care, reduction in hospital complications (e.g. readmissions), or improvement in patient outcomes. The VOI approach provides a straightforward way of articulating the "bang for your buck" for any given initiative. For example, a tele-ICU program that cost $700,000 annually may demonstrate an improvement in mortality statistics (actual vs. predicted), resulting in 50 lives saved in one year. The VOI statement would be that for every $14,000 invested in tele-ICU, a life was saved. In addition, secondary impacts can be included in the VOI equation to capture peripheral effects of the service. For the tele-ICU example, secondary impacts may include an improvement in case mix index, a decrease in length of hospital stay, or an increase in ICU nurse retention.

5.6 Funding from alternative sources

As telehealth offers the opportunity to mitigate barriers to accessing care, there are often many stakeholders interested in leveraging the opportunity to improve the health of underserved communities and other shared societal benefits. The health system's commitment to the community may provide opportunities for funding and resource allocation. Community philanthropy, government agencies, and non-profit agencies may likewise have opportunities to provide support outside of the traditional healthcare infrastructure. For programs seeking to provide the largest scope of change in healthcare access through innovation, these alternative sources of funding may offer the largest opportunities in the early stages of the program's maturity.

5.7 Billing compliance

Telehealth reimbursement policies can vary and continue to evolve rapidly. Telehealth services are vetted by billing compliance professionals to assess current payor polices and recommend the most profitable, compliant billing codes. Collaborating with billing compliance and revenue cycle personnel during the Development phase will increase the likelihood of improving the capture of professional billing revenue. Many third-party payor telehealth policies only recognize specific "eligible services" (i.e. which codes will be reimbursed), "eligible providers" (i.e. who can be reimbursed for services) and "eligible sites" (i.e. the place of service where patients must be in order to qualify for reimbursement). With telehealth reimbursement policies changing rapidly, it is beneficial to have at least an annual review of telehealth billing practices to ensure both compliance and optimal revenue generation.

6 | Telehealth for efficient, effective care

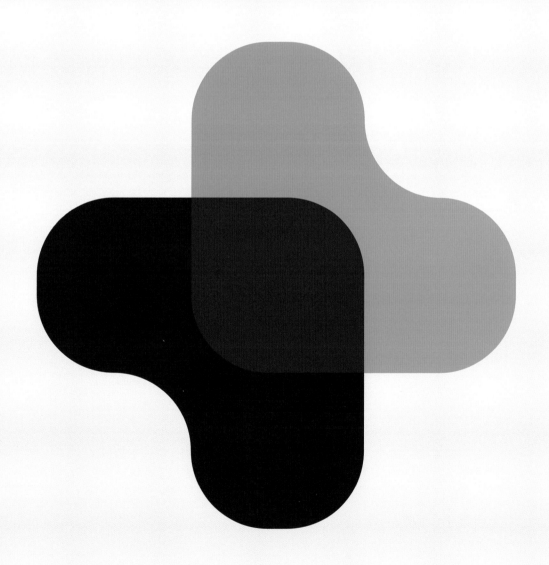

The Strategy phase of TSIM defines the goals, value, and scope of the service. One overarching theme governs these three actions: telehealth services should not simply replicate traditional care over distance using technology, but should enhance the efficiency of the system while not sacrificing effective clinical care. If the current inefficient delivery of care is replicated, the full potential of telehealth will never be realized. When developing telehealth services, one should focus on the clinical goals of care, and after identifying the primary value for the service, the technology can be leveraged to identify new ways to redesign the workflow in a more efficient, effective way to achieve those goals.

While in-person care offers opportunities for comprehensive assessments at a single moment, telehealth offers more opportunities to leverage care along the continuum through a sequence of contacts with a patient over time, as contact is generally more convenient for both the patient and the provider. Additionally, telehealth models have the opportunity to create new provider efficiencies and allow patients to receive acute care in the comfort of their own homes. Finally, emerging care delivery models, leveraging artificial intelligence, will revolutionize the clinical quality and delivery of care.

These new technologies can support clinical transformation, but clinical transformation does not occur at the point of technology procurement. It is achieved at the intersection of clinical, technical, and business personnel collaborating to create innovative and sustainable telehealth models. TSIM supports the development and implementation of these new models of efficient care delivery.

6.1 Focusing on clinical goals of care

When developing a telehealth service, it is important to keep the clinical goals at the forefront. The most successful telehealth programs gravitate towards the resolution of specific care goals, such as with telestroke, in which the care team is managing discrete decisions on a care pathway. Such focused decisions can be handled well with technology to guide collaborative teams over distance. This is in contrast to the typical approach to in-person care, in which the team tries to maximize the relatively rare opportunity to engage a patient and be as comprehensive as possible in the limited time available. While the previous in-person processes may not consider the advantages that are specific to telehealth, acknowledging and accepting these differences illuminate the opportunity for clinical transformation.

Another advantage to keeping the telehealth strategy focused on the clinical goals of care is that it avoids the common pitfall of designing the programs around the technology itself. A telehealth pitfall is distraction by the novelty of the technology at the expense of thoughtful care goals, which jeopardizes the overall strategic purpose. Developing governance structures around technologies, and using these structures to identify standard choices that can be periodically updated as technology evolves, often helps to avoid this common hazard. Caution must be taken to ensure that these processes do not limit long-term effectiveness and reduce the ability to synergize multiple interventions (telehealth or not) with common goals.

6.2 Identifying the primary value

Technological innovations applied in the healthcare setting often bring forth many potential opportunities for improvement in healthcare delivery. While this is exciting, traditional return-on-investment formulas typically do not capture the overall value of a telehealth service, and in order for a telehealth service to have the best chance of success, it is beneficial to recognize the most important reason for its innovation. In other words, it is important to identify the primary value that the program will provide (see Table 6.1). A telehealth program may well have multiple impacts and different quality, cost, and health improvement metrics, but these may be hard to achieve without specifically identifying the most important of these and designing and aligning the resources towards this targeted goal.

Table 6.1 Examples of primary value drivers

Primary value	Primary intent	Example service
Contracted care	To provide consistent contractual revenue	Telestroke
Primary care integration	To support the primary care model with telehealth resources	Nutritional telecounseling
Health equity	To reduce a health inequity	School-based telehealth
Access to care	To establish new access points of care	Regional telehealth clinics
Convenient care	To improve the convenience of care for patients	Ambulatory telehealth visits
Cost avoidance	To mitigate the risk of financial penalties or costs	Post-discharge RPM
Quality and safety	To improve the quality and/or safety of patient care	Telesitter

The primary value can establish a "North Star" that a telehealth program can align and realign to over a trajectory of time. It allows for a quantifiable goal, aids in business planning and sustainability tactics, and can provide strong messaging and sense of responsiveness to key stakeholders.

An honest assessment of where a program is headed once at scale may involve shifting a primary target or value case. For example, a program may be set up to benefit an underserved population, but may also be able to show progress in improving clinical service and/or hospital finances. Conversely, if the program turns out to require an unintended level of commitment from the team involved, or its intended value is not demonstrable as it achieves scale, the primary value may need to be adjusted to maintain commitment from appropriate stakeholders. An example of this is when a program brings some benefit to a high-risk patient population but not necessarily financial value to the health system. The institutions involved may continue to deem the program worthwhile to continue if the true value is well articulated. In this case, the primary value case has become that of service to the underserved population or a decrease in the health equity gap, and the stakeholders are now investors towards that particular goal.

6.3 Care along the continuum

Telehealth technologies can be strategically used to encourage patient engagement over time and across the continuum of care. Integrating digital care along the continuum can serve as a common thread throughout the patient journey, establishing a more holistic patient experience. Hybrid care models that integrate telehealth with in-person care at key points along the continuum can create new efficiencies and provide more convenient care. Digital care along the continuum provides a foundation for how best to interact with patients based upon their healthcare needs and their natural level of engagement.

At the most basic level, the "generally well" patient population can be engaged through asynchronous educational or health surveillance reminders. Patients who have engaged through a virtual care platform, or patient portal, for convenience purposes during times of minor acute illness may also fall into this category when reminders or screenings are then sent back to them.

Patient populations who have been determined to be at risk for a certain diagnosis may fall into a higher level of care which may include asynchronous screenings to detect changes in their symptoms over time and provide access to early diagnosis and treatment options. Examples of this type of intervention might be post-traumatic stress disorder screenings for patients who have experienced trauma, peripartum depression screenings for childbearing women, or post-operative questionnaires to detect surgical complications.

Lastly, patients who have been diagnosed with a chronic disease may be prescribed an RPM program in order to increase their engagement in managing their own health. These interventions are typically asynchronous and include both physiological metrics and patient-reported outcomes that allow the healthcare team to make more timely adjustments to the care plan. Examples of these technologies include diabetes, hypertension and heart failure RPM programs.

All of these digital approaches along the care continuum are meant to be additive to traditional in-person care. This level of access, in which providers can be digitally present in their patients' daily lives, can transform the continuum of care such that patients are able to conveniently interact with the healthcare system no matter what their health status or level of interest may be.

6.4 Provider care efficiencies

Many clinical specialties are experiencing nationwide provider shortages, but new telehealth delivery models can create efficiencies in the delivery of care.[42] Early in the global COVID-19 pandemic, there were reports of national telehealth companies that used synchronous (i.e. phone and video) technologies having long wait times and substantial struggles due to the increased demand for online services. This traditional (replication of care) approach using phone or video can result in the virtual visit mirroring the typical 15-minute length of an in-person visit. In contrast, asynchronous technology solutions have been able to take that same encounter down to an 89-second clinical decision through intelligent patient intake logic, improving provider efficiency and helping health systems to achieve scale.[43]

RPM and mHealth delivery models can also increase provider efficiencies. For example, diabetic RPM programs can allow a nurse to monitor hundreds of patients at a time. Through intelligent dashboarding of the data, the RPM nurse can focus on those patients who have significantly abnormal glucose values or vital signs specific to the clinical parameters established by their physician. Diabetic RPM programs have also demonstrated significant improvements in medication adherence and decreased hemoglobin A1C levels, resulting in significant healthcare cost savings.[44]

6.5 Hospital at home

New hospital-at-home telehealth models enable healthcare organizations to create virtual beds without ever laying a brick.[45] A hospital-at-home delivery model allows patients to receive care in the comfort of their own home while being monitored by hospital support staff using telehealth and other digital health applications. While hospital-at-home models have been well established in other countries, their adoption in the US has been slow, mainly due to third-party payors offering limited reimbursement for care delivered into the home. However, studies have shown that hospital-at-home models can reduce costs, increase patient satisfaction, and decrease risk for some patient complications (e.g. delirium).

During the peak of the global pandemic, many healthcare organizations used the hospital-at-home model to remotely monitor patients with COVID-19.[46] This RPM model provided medical support to isolated patients and helped mitigate additional exposure risks. In addition, through asynchronous symptom tracking, the medical staff were able to safely escalate patients into higher levels of care when needed. As reimbursement payments continue to shift towards value-based care, hospital-at-home delivery models are expected to become more evident throughout the US.

6.6 Emerging care delivery models

Emerging care delivery models that leverage artificial intelligence (AI) and related technologies are becoming more prevalent in healthcare.[47] AI is a collection of different types of technologies such as machine learning, natural language processing, and robotics. As its name implies, machine learning is the use of AI to enable technology systems to learn and improve from experience without explicit programming. Such systems learn and become more precise when provided with larger volumes of data.

Machine learning (ML) has demonstrated success in identifying clinically relevant features in radiologic images (e.g. identifying tumors) and holds significant promise in the healthcare industry. Natural language processing (NLP) combines linguistics and AI to help machines process and understand the human language in various contexts through pattern recognition in speech and written text. During the global pandemic, researchers gathered data from a virtual urgent care asynchronous technology solution and used NLP to identify that the words "smell," "taste," "sense," and "lost" were used at a much higher frequency with patients who eventually tested positive for COVID-19. The result of this study was that the asynchronous technology solution was modified to include specific questions related to loss of sense of taste and smell.[48] Finally, robotics can provide an increase in medical procedural precision and is used frequently in many surgical procedures. While these emerging care delivery models may vary, the TSIM framework provides a standardized clinical transformation approach to assess for applicability and ensure that there is a process to integrate them into the traditional system.

7 | Outcomes planning

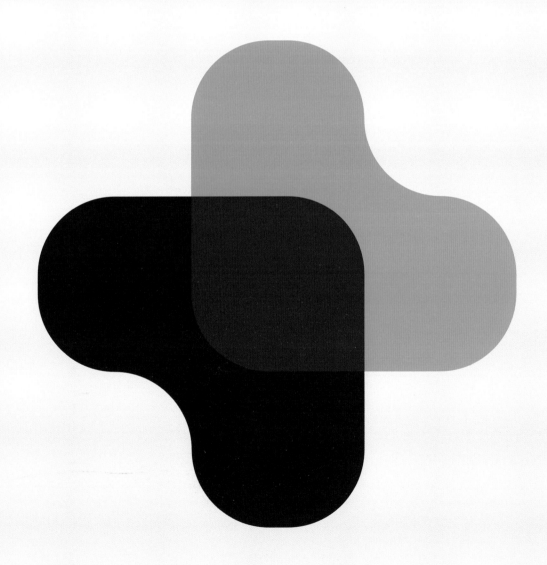

7.1 Defining metrics of success

In alignment with the telehealth service's primary value, it is beneficial to identify metrics that will be tracked to assess the success of the service being developed. If metrics of success are not clearly defined and collectively agreed to within Strategy, different stakeholders may have different perspectives on what success looks like, and the disjointed views can have a significant negative impact on maturing a program. The 2017 final report by the National Quality Forum (NQF), "Creating a framework to support measure development for telehealth," serves as an excellent guide and classifies success metrics into the following domains: access to care, financial impact/cost, experience, and effectiveness.[49] These high-level domains can be broken down further into subdomains (see Table 7.1). The NQF framework provides an outline to define standardized telehealth metrics (i.e. key performance indicators) that are appropriate for the locally developed services.

Table 7.1 NQF's telehealth measurement framework

Domain	Subdomain(s)
Access to care	Access for patient, family, and/or caregiver Access for care team Access for information
Financial impact/cost	Financial impact to patient, family, and/or caregiver Financial impact to care team Financial impact to health system or payor Financial impact to society
Experience	Patient, family, and/or caregiver experience Care team member experience Community experience
Effectiveness	System effectiveness Clinical effectiveness Operational effectiveness Technical effectiveness

7.2 Standardized telehealth metrics

7.2.1 Utilization metric

Utilization is defined as the number of telehealth interactions that are completed in a given time period. A telehealth interaction is a single virtual encounter or transfer of medical information over distance for the benefit of the patient. Telehealth interactions are monitored as an aggregate total and also broken down into their respective modes of delivery (e.g. synchronous, RPM). By monitoring telehealth interactions, a healthcare organization can assess the adoption level of the service and implement changes within the Continuous Quality Improvement phase if utilization is not achieving original projections for the service.

7.2.2 Patient and provider experience metrics

The experience of the people involved in the telehealth encounter (i.e. patients and providers) is continuously evaluated to monitor the user-friendliness of the service. An effective and simple measurement tool to assess patient and provider experience is the Net Promoter Score (NPS). This is used across many industries as a customer loyalty and satisfaction metric, and is based on a simple question regarding the customer's likelihood to recommend a company or product. The NPS formula accounts for promoters, passives, and detractors, and a final NPS score is calculated to assess the users' experience with the telehealth service (see Table 7.2).

An example of a patient experience question is "On a scale of 0 to 10, how likely are you to recommend this telehealth service to a friend?" For provider experience, healthcare organizations can ask "On a scale of 0 to 10, how likely are you to recommend the use of this telehealth service to a colleague?" Because many telehealth services are provider-to-provider based, it is very beneficial to assess perspectives of both consulting and referring providers. When the trend of a score changes significantly, it is recommended to conduct deeper-dive interviews to better understand what is impacting the service so issues can be resolved (negative impacts) or shared as best practice (positive impacts).

Table 7.2 Net Promoter Score for assessing telehealth services[50]

User category	Category score	User description
Promoters	Score of 9 or 10	The most loyal and satisfied users of the service
Passives	Score of 7 or 8	Users who felt neutral about their experience
Detractors	Score of 0 to 6	Users who had a bad experience with the service and are most likely to tell others about it

Net Promoter Score = % promoters – % detractors

Scores range from –100 to 100

- Scores from –100 to 0 mean that most users are having a bad experience.
- Scores from 1 to 30 indicate that slightly more users are having a good experience than bad experience, but opportunities for improvement are evident.
- Scores from 31 to 50 make up a normal range that demonstrates quality user experience.
- Scores from 51 to 70 demonstrate a higher-than-average user experience.
- Scores from 71 to 100 validate a "best-in-class" user experience.

7.2.3 Quality of care delivery metrics

Quality of care delivery metrics can be divided into two categories: the efficiency of care delivery and the clinical effectiveness of care delivered. The efficiency of care delivery metrics is typically time- or volume-based metrics. These process metrics allow a healthcare organization to assess the performance of the delivery of the telehealth service. Examples of efficiency of care delivery process measures include provider response times, no-show rates, and time to scheduled consult. These measures help assess the delivery of the service and identify areas for improvement.

Metrics that assess the clinical effectiveness of care delivery focus on clinical outcomes that are specific to the type of specialty being delivered. Examples of clinical effectiveness quality metrics include "door-to-needle" times (telestroke), antibiotic stewardship (infectious disease consultations), and fall reductions (telesitter). Many telehealth services may also have more long-term (downstream) quality metrics to monitor, such as a reduction in emergency room visits for pediatric asthmatic patients (school-based telehealth), lowering A1C levels (diabetic RPM), or decreased mortality rate (tele-ICU). Clinical champions are essential for identifying key quality of care metrics relevant to the telehealth service being developed.

7.2.4 Technical reliability metric

Assessing the technical reliability of the telehealth platform on a continuous basis is imperative. If its reliability is not adequate, this can negatively impact all other performance measures. Providers and patients need to trust that the encounter will work effectively for them at the point of the connection. Examples of telehealth platform reliability metrics include uptime/availability, number of technical incidents, and mean time to recover/repair (MTTR). Technical reliability metrics should be monitored, and minimally acceptable requirements established and enforced with technology personnel and telehealth technology vendors.

7.2.5 Sustainability metric

Sustainability can be monitored via a financial metric and/or a primary value metric. For scaled telehealth services in more traditional business models (e.g. hospital support services), profit margin is a standard metric to assess the financial sustainability of a service. To calculate a telehealth service's net profit margin, which is expressed as a percentage, simply subtract cost from revenue (i.e. net income) and divide by the revenue (see below).[51]

$$\text{Net profit margin} = (\text{revenue} - \text{cost}) \div \text{revenue}$$

Since telehealth often offers a VOI that sometimes differs from the traditional return on investment, sustainability may depend on the primary value of the service. To calculate the VOI, the financial investment made for the service is divided into the impact (see below). Utilization and clinical effectiveness can be used to determine the impact of the telehealth service.

$$\text{Value on investment} = \text{impact} \div \text{investment}$$

Establishing financial or value metrics will help telehealth departments have honest discussions about their time and effort as business models for telehealth services continue to evolve. Sustainability of telehealth services can be a significant weakness for telehealth programs, but successful, sustainable services are achievable. Identifying the sustainability metric(s) in Strategy with key stakeholders, and developing a report to track the service's performance, allows better visibility of challenges and an opportunity for timely strategic decisions as the service and payment policies continue to evolve.

7.3 Performance metric maturity model

A series of short-, medium-, and long-term outcomes can be applied that align with the maturity of the program and serve to guide its direction towards the intended primary value outcome (see Table 7.3). Process-level metrics are used initially as short-term goals. As programs grow, these are followed by medium-term goals and impacts related to the growth and scope of the program. Finally, health system and population level impacts are major long-term outcomes. Establishing a performance metric maturity model early will set the vision for the team, while simultaneously outlining a pathway to achieve those long-term goals.

Table 7.3 Performance metric maturity model

Category	Short term	Medium term	Long term
Utilization	Encounter volume	Encounters measured against expected	Encounters as proportion of volume needed for intended impact
Effectiveness	User satisfaction	Short-term clinical impact and process measures	Longer-term health and health system impact
Sustainability	Support cost and associated revenues	Expanded business planning	Operating margin and downstream revenues

8 | TSIM phases: Pipeline and Strategy

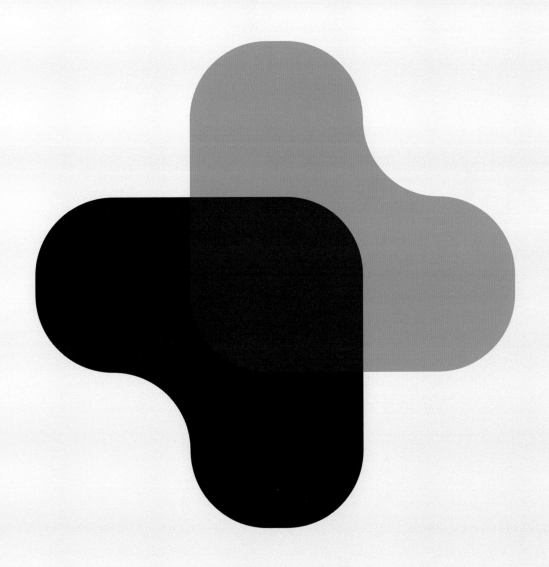

8.1 Pipeline (pre-Strategy phase)

As new ideas for telehealth services arise, it is beneficial to have a formalized process to submit and receive these requests in a structured manner (see Figure 8.1). Thus, the Pipeline phase organizes and manages the flow of service development requests. Stakeholders, from clinical staff to hospital administrators armed with new applications of telehealth in their field of interest, can be directed to an online telehealth idea submission portal.

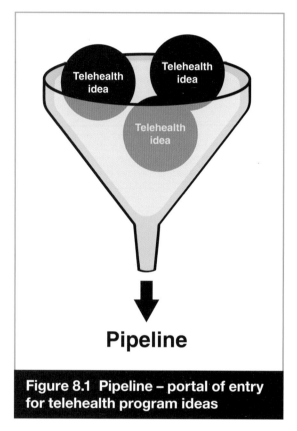

Figure 8.1 Pipeline – portal of entry for telehealth program ideas

This step involves a very brief written introduction to the telehealth idea, including the clinical specialty, the population the service is intended to serve, the problem it will solve, and a high-level concept of how it will be delivered. A small leadership team can then assess the idea for strategic alignment, potential financial support, and technical feasibility. The local health system identifies the most appropriate leadership team, ideally two or three people, to conduct this initial assessment. The team should be cognizant of the organizational strategic plan, existing telehealth technology and funding resources, and team capacity to develop the new ideas.

While it may seem cumbersome to have this initial screen, it can save significant time and resources while ensuring telehealth staff are focused on the ideas that are most likely to come to fruition. Additionally, this phase gives both the leadership and support teams an idea of the volume of requests and which proposals to anticipate are moving into later phases. If an idea does not align with the current strategy or the necessary resources are not available, the service will not be developed, but it may be modified or deferred until a later date. When the new idea has strategic alignment and resources are available to support its development, it is advanced into the Strategy phase, and a formal intake of the service idea is initiated.

8.2 Strategy phase

The Strategy phase is central to the TSIM framework (see Figure 8.2). The key priorities of Strategy are focused on articulating the problem(s) the telehealth service is intended to solve, defining the overall goals and success metrics of the care to be delivered, and identifying the primary value that the program adds to the system. It is at this juncture where it is important to avoid reverting to the previous in-person processes and focus instead on the goals of the innovation. By "wiping clean" the slate of how care has traditionally been delivered, one can reimagine a model of care delivery where patients and providers have enhanced access to connect over time. Overall, the process achieves some predetermined value and provides efficiencies in care delivery. Once the goals of care and the value case are defined, the scope of the program can then take shape, with these overarching principles serving as parameters.

After the idea is vetted and cleared to advance from Pipeline, the telehealth team takes a structured approach to ensure standard information is collected, resources are allocated relative to strategic priorities, and performance metrics are identified. In addition, technology and timeline projections are made, and the final scope is clearly defined and approved within a service charter. Practical elements such as legal, compliance, capacities of resources, and technology are all considered at a high level, with the specific operational details addressed in the Development phase.

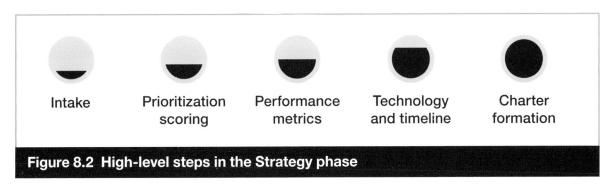

| Intake | Prioritization scoring | Performance metrics | Technology and timeline | Charter formation |

Figure 8.2 High-level steps in the Strategy phase

8.3 Intake process

The progression from an innovative telehealth service idea to a clearly defined strategy can be a daunting task, but it is not necessary to have all the strategic elements fleshed out in this first step. However, key elements of the strategy are articulated up front to guide decisions and inform eventual elements within the Development phase to follow. A standard intake form, retrieved through an interview with the requestor, is completed at the beginning of Strategy (see Table 8.1).

This standardized approach documents the narrative of the most important guiding strategic elements and provides the early boundaries of creating a clearly defined scope. It also directs the focused collection of information needed to outline the goals and primary value of the service. The vision articulated during this intake process may shift as the service goes through stages of TSIM, and the team may find it healthy to review the intake form periodically as strategic decisions are made.

Table 8.1 Sample intake form

Date	August 28, 2021
Telehealth service idea	Inpatient Teleneurology
Service requestor	Tiffany Schroeder, VP of Neurology Services
Service line	Neurology
Who will be the executive champion?	Tiffany Schroeder, VP of Neurology Services
Who will be the clinical champion(s)?	Dr. Brooklyn Rae, Dr. Cecilia Rose, Dr. Scarlett Raine
Define the scope of the service	The Inpatient Teleneurology service will provide scheduled telehealth consultations for general neurological conditions at partnering hospitals
What problem is being solved via telehealth?	This service will improve access to expert neurology care that is limited or not available in many community hospitals
What condition(s) will be treated?	General neurological conditions (e.g. stroke follow-up, seizures)
When will the service be available?	Scheduled consultations available from 8:00 a.m. to 5:00 p.m., seven days a week
Who will be the consulting providers?	Neurologists
Where will the patients be located?	Hospitals – inpatient
How will success of the service be measured?	The goal is to partner with enough hospitals to fill a full day's schedule within six months after go-live to achieve a positive net profit margin
What is the business model or pathway to sustainability?	Hospitals will be charged for access to the service; professional billing will be submitted for each encounter
What workflow will be used?	Scheduled workflow
What telehealth modality will be used? Other tech requirements?	Real-time synchronous video encounters, delivered on a cart-based solution with pan-tilt-zoom; telehealth software with image sharing
Expected primary value	Contracted care – hospital support service

8.4 Prioritization scoring

The process of scoring a new request or idea with a standardized prioritization tool assists the team in its work management. In addition, it helps to ensure that the services have a high likelihood of succeeding when they enter the subsequent TSIM phases. An example approach to strategic scoring includes three main categories: implementation support, potential impact, and sustainability (see Table 8.2).

Table 8.2 Example of prioritization scoring criteria

Instructions:

- The first column lists the three main categories to be evaluated.
- There are three domains for each category, shown in the second column.
- Use the third column to rate each domain from a score of 1 (lowest) to 4 (highest).
- Calculate the total priority score by adding all of the domain scores together. The highest possible score is 36.

Category	Domain	Scoring criteria
Implementation support	Strategic alignment	4) Addresses objectives/needs of the enterprise strategic plan
		3) Addresses objectives/needs of the clinical department's strategic plan
		2) Considered priority of the clinical division
		1) Has clinical leadership's support
	Provider champion(s)	4) Multiple providers engaged
		3) Single provider engaged
		2) Provider champion identified
		1) No provider champion identified
	Provider capacity	4) Adequate capacity to implement and expand the service
		3) Adequate capacity to implement the service
		2) Adequate capacity to pilot the service
		1) Need to strategically hire to pilot the service
Potential impact	Total cost of care	4) Service is expected to have a significant reduction in total cost of care
		3) Service is expected to have a moderate reduction in total cost of care
		2) Service is expected to have a minimal reduction in total cost of care
		1) Service is not expected to reduce the total cost of care

Table continues

Table 8.2 *continued*

Potential impact *continued*	Quality	4) Service is projected to significantly improve quality outcomes
		3) Service is projected to have a moderate improvement in quality outcomes
		2) Service is projected to have a minimal improvement in quality outcomes
		1) Service is not projected to improve quality outcomes
	Access to care	4) Service is projected to significantly increase access to care for a target patient population
		3) Service is projected to make a moderate improvement in accessing care for the overall population
		2) Service is projected to make a slight improvement in accessing care
		1) Service is not expected to increase access to care
Sustainability	Potential market reach	4) Service has potential to serve a national market
		3) Service has potential to serve a region of the national market
		2) Service has potential to serve the statewide population
		1) Service is likely limited to serving the local region
	Financial analysis	4) Proven business model with a significant ROI
		3) New business model with a significant projected ROI
		2) Business model with a minimal/moderately projected ROI
		1) Business model has substantial sustainability risks
	Current demand	4) Service is in high demand with patients and/or referring sites
		3) Service has moderate level of demand with patients and/or referring sites
		2) Service has interest expressed by potential patients and/or referring sites
		1) Interest/demand for service is unknown
Total priority score =		

8.4.1 Prioritizing scoring – implementation support

Implementation support is the first category, which incorporates key factors that impact the success of developing and implementing the service (i.e. internal potential readiness). This category asks the team to review the alignment with the organizational strategic plan, the commitment of a provider champion, and the capacity of clinical staffing available to grow the service if developed. When new telehealth initiatives align with existing organizational strategy, the synergistic efforts of complementary initiatives and executive leadership support provide an optimal environment for a telehealth service to succeed.

A provider champion is the dedicated clinical leader of the telehealth service. The provider champion can represent the clinical needs of their respective division or department, and their leadership and advocacy will be imperative in order to navigate the significant change management steps required to transform care delivery. Sometimes telehealth ideas come from external demand or administrative leadership, and the clinical capacity is not available to implement the service. Accounting for those provider capacity constraints can save health systems substantial time when deciding to allocate resources for a particular telehealth initiative.

8.4.2 Prioritizing scoring – potential impact

The second category projects the potential impact of the service across the domains of total cost of care, quality, and access to care. As the healthcare industry is in a transformational period, with a continued focus on addressing the Institute for Healthcare Improvement's Triple Aim,[52] telehealth services are well positioned to create new efficiencies within the care delivery system, and the second category of the scoring tool assesses the potential impact of these earned efficiencies. The telehealth service is evaluated by projecting its potential impact on total cost of care, quality, and access to care. While the assessment of potential impact lends itself to the most subjectivity, stopping to reflect on what the service is intended to accomplish is a valuable exercise and aligns with associated outcomes planning.

8.4.3 Prioritizing scoring – sustainability

The final category asks the team to consider the sustainability of the service with a high-level review of potential market reach, financial analysis, and current demand. The potential market reach is intended to understand the breadth of a market the service could potentially serve (e.g. local, regional, national). The finance analysis helps assess the maturity of the business planning, with a preference for telehealth models that have already demonstrated financial success. Finally, while empiric data may suggest a need for a particular telehealth service, the actual demand for the service may be lagging. Unless there is clear demand for the service from potential customers, utilization will suffer.

8.5 Performance metrics identified

Within the Strategy phase, metrics and outcomes are identified that will define the success of the telehealth service. To create standardization across telehealth services and aid in performance tracking, it is helpful to establish standardized telehealth performance metrics (i.e. key performance indicators, or KPIs) that can track the progress of the service from initial go-live through all stages of telehealth program maturity (see Table 8.3). Reviewing these KPI metrics periodically for all programs will lead to a systematic approach to tracking success and quality and give guidance to improvement processes. Defining performance metrics early can help inform the system build needed to collect these metrics once the program has gone live and set expectations going forward. Specific financial and process metrics will be determined by the program, its goals, the primary value case, and the respective stakeholders.

As with all healthcare initiatives, a sustainability plan or business model is an essential part of planning. With innovations in the healthcare space, this can be complicated, as the payment models are typically designed for the traditional FFS reimbursement model that the innovation is seeking to alter. Considering direct, indirect, and alternative sources of financial support, financial metrics are established to continuously monitor the service's actual performance in relation to what was initially projected. The telehealth service will initially be assessed through the use of process, quality, and financial metrics for the purpose of program implementation and continuous improvement, and will eventually evolve into a longer-term evaluation arm for research and ultimate success evaluation.

Table 8.3 **Examples of standardized telehealth performance metrics**

Metric	Explanation
Utilization	The total number of telehealth interactions that are completed in a given time period
Provider experience	Net Promoter Score to assess the experience of the providers
Patient experience	Net Promoter Score to assess the experience of the patients
Quality of care delivery	Efficiency and/or clinical effectiveness of care delivery
Reliability	A metric to assess the technical reliability of the service
Sustainability	A financial metric to assess pathway to sustainability

8.6 Technology

While a full and final assessment on selecting the appropriate telehealth technologies for the service will occur in Development, initial strategic implications can be articulated within Strategy to assist in essential early planning. As telehealth technologies become increasingly common, it is likely that the tools available to the team will be dictated by those that are available from the institution or the stakeholders involved. Sorting through these technological options includes defining the individuals or care teams who are intended to interact, what clinical elements are needed to influence management decisions, and at what frequency the information is intended to be available. Additionally, the sustainability plan associated with the program may influence whether the communication technologies will be limited by billing compliance factors.

It is in the Strategy phase of TSIM where the team considers technology choices beyond using video to replicate the traditional encounter. Returning to the telehealth service's stated goals and strategy can help with this process. Unfortunately, in the traditional FFS reimbursement system, technology choices are often dictated by billing compliance rules as opposed to optimal clinical efficiency and effectiveness. Allowances in the sustainability planning to take advantage of added efficiencies of care and downstream revenues will serve to liberalize the technology options that can be considered.

In the Strategy phase, it is also beneficial to begin to address the core decision related to integrations with existing electronic health systems. Reviewing which integrations are available, which are necessary, and which may be burdensome can help the team move forward in Development with a common understanding of the intended functioning of the technology and resources needed.

A final, and perhaps the most important, consideration related to technology during Strategy is to have a clear understanding of the impact of the accessibility and usability of the technologies to the users. Ease of use can become the primary limiting factor to the telehealth service, and should be considered prominently with technology choices. Factors influencing ease of use depend on adequate training in the care setting, and the users' digital literacy and level of engagement. This is increasingly important with the growth of telehealth. As more patient-facing telehealth technologies are deployed rapidly across an enterprise, there is limited ability to provide training, a wider range of digital literacy, and a spectrum of user engagement that often trends lower in those most in need, such as underserved populations.

8.7 Timeline projections

An additional assessment is made regarding resource allocation and anticipated critical timeline factors that may affect service development. While these practical elements may not be part of the scoring criteria, they are likely to influence the ability to progress the service, and at a minimum are used to set realistic expectations for all relevant stakeholders. Some examples of factors that may lengthen the time to go-live include obtaining state medical licenses, executing legal agreements, receiving credentialing approval, configuring and/or integrating technology, and designing a new telehealth workflow that has not been locally demonstrated yet. Armed with the initial score, information about resource allocation, and critical timeline implications, the telehealth team can then prioritize the program among the others in its current portfolio and establish an initial implementation timeline.

8.8 Service charter formation

With the scope clearly defined and metrics identified, a telehealth service development coordinator is assigned as the accountable owner for the completion of the service charter document and to navigate the service through the Development phase. The service charter document uses the information gathered in the intake process, together with the feedback obtained through the subsequent Strategy discussions, to clearly define the scope of the service. This phase involves considering the scale of the service needed to achieve the intended outcomes, the capacity of the service providers, the availability of supporting resources (e.g. nursing, telepresenters), and legal and compliance parameters.

While completing the service charter document, it is important to have a clearly articulated focus and to specify the care delivery problem or opportunity that is being addressed. At this point, the concept of a high-level clinical workflow and planned technological endpoints is documented, with the understanding that those elements may be modified once the service reaches the Development phase. Initial business or sustainability plans are established based on the primary value case and process metrics. In addition, short-, medium-, and long-term metrics of success are established. It is reasonable to assume that the initiative will not have all of the specific decisions resolved, as that comes later in the Development phase, but the team should understand the intended scope and constraints in order to set reasonable expectations and balance the initiative against other institutional priorities.

It is important to distribute the final version of the service charter through an internal brief to both complete the communication loop with the initial requestor and inform the project stakeholders who will be engaged within the Development phase. This internal brief may be a meeting or an email communication to the relevant stakeholders that the telehealth service will be entering the Development phase. At the time of this communication, the telehealth coordinator who has been assigned as the accountable owner presents the service charter document and solicits any final questions or clarifications needed for the team prior to progressing into the Development phase.

9 | TSIM phase: Development

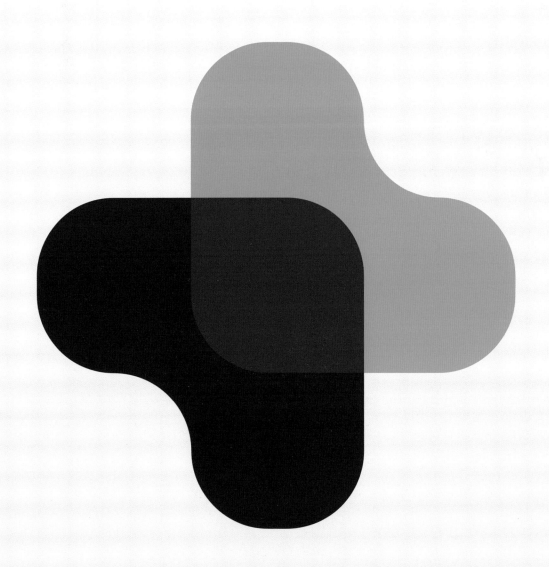

9.1 Introduction

After the service charter is finalized, the Development phase is initiated and the telehealth service is created, based on the scope defined in the Strategy phase. Development is one of the most complex phases to navigate. It is very project management heavy, with numerous tasks to complete that span over a vast array of stakeholders across many clinical, operational, and technical departments. To ensure coordination of all of the tasks that need to be completed, a Development pre-check meeting is scheduled to bring all of the relevant members of the project team together to review the scope of the telehealth service. Examples of the stakeholders engaged within the Development phase include, but are not limited to, clinical champions, informaticists, IT personnel, legal, billing compliance, revenue cycle, scheduling, credentialing, risk management, information security, and procurement.

TSIM establishes the following four core Development pathways to navigate: (1) clinical, (2) technology, (3) legal and regulatory, and (4) outcomes (see Figure 9.1). The tasks that need to be completed will depend on many different factors, such as the type of service and the location setting in which the service will be delivered. Once all of the tasks have been completed within the four Development pathways, the telehealth project team comes together at the launch status brief (LSB) meeting to set a projected go-live date and transition into the Implementation phase.

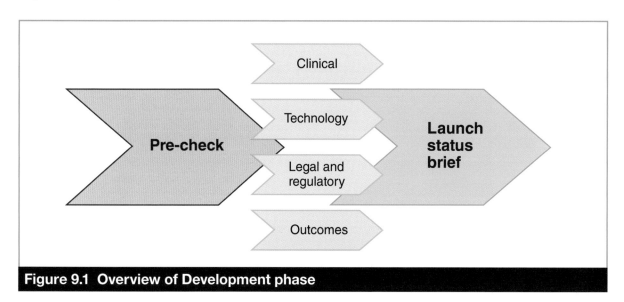

Figure 9.1 Overview of Development phase

9.2 Development pre-check

The process of developing telehealth services is not linear across these pathways, and there can be numerous interconnected dependencies. Asking standardized questions that address each Development pathway helps identify what tasks will need to be completed (see Table 9.1). It is within this meeting that assignments are provided so it is clear who is accountable and responsible for each task. In addition, key stakeholders are identified for specific tasks that they are to be consulted on or about which they need to be kept informed.

Table 9.1 Guide for pre-check meeting

Development pathway	Questions to review in development pre-check meeting
Clinical	What is the ideal clinical workflow of the telehealth service? What system development and/or configurations are needed to support the clinical workflow? What type of scheduling support is required to support the service? What training will be required, and what educational/training resources need to be created?
Technology	Will telehealth technology need to be purchased? If new technology will be procured, what are the clinical needs, operational functionality, and technical requirements for the telehealth platform or device? What technical support is needed to implement and maintain service expectations?
Legal and regulatory	What are the legal and regulatory obligations that should be considered for the service? Will this service need contracts with any third parties? Are the providers already licensed and credentialed, and do they have appropriate malpractice insurance coverage?
Outcomes	How will the success of the telehealth service be measured? What data sources will serve as the "source of truth" for outcomes? How will data reports be validated?

9.3 Clinical pathway

The clinical pathway of the Development phase is when the clinical workflow is drafted and finalized, and operational plans and protocols are created to support the new service. Having a clear and efficient clinical workflow for the telehealth service is one of the most important tasks in all of TSIM. In order to design the integration of telehealth into the traditional delivery system, it is imperative to understand the healthcare team's current clinical workflow. Touring and shadowing in the clinical areas where the provider will conduct the telehealth service, as well as where the patient will be located, can be a useful exercise. This experience will provide the opportunity to better understand the current clinical environment and all of its nuances prior to developing the service.

9.3.1 Clinical workflows

Clinical workflows will differ depending on a variety of factors including the condition(s) being addressed, type of provider, and patient location. It is essential to have the clinical champion heavily engaged with the development of the clinical workflow. The two foundational workflows for synchronous interactions are an "on-demand" and a "scheduled" workflow. The on-demand workflow is for when a clinical provider must be immediately available to respond (e.g. telestroke). A scheduled workflow is when a patient is scheduled for a telehealth encounter sometime in the future (e.g. ambulatory care). A swim lane diagram can be a useful tool to design a clinical workflow and designate roles and responsibilities among the care team members (see Figure 9.2). Standardizing workflows for each care setting will help mitigate operational and technical support issues.

During the creation of the clinical workflow, decisions on documentation and billing will be finalized, informed by the support of legal and billing compliance experts. Once the workflow is drafted, it is important that all relevant stakeholders approve a finalized version. This step helps ensure that clinical, operational, and technical staff are given the opportunity to review the workflow, provide feedback on it, and approve the final version. The new workflow will disrupt the traditional delivery of care in both anticipated and unanticipated ways, and securing early buy-in is essential in effectively navigating change management throughout the Implementation phase.

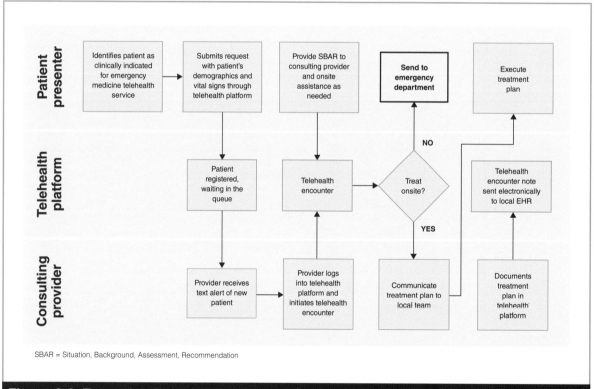

SBAR = Situation, Background, Assessment, Recommendation

Figure 9.2 Example of an emergency medicine telehealth service workflow

9.3.2 Clinical and operational protocols

Once the workflow for the telehealth service has been approved by the necessary stakeholders, additional elements are considered for the collaborating (patient originating) site to align with the telehealth workflow. For example, in a setting such as a hospital, new clinical order sets, policies, and/or protocols may need to be created to support the new telehealth service. Guidelines are established on how to handle patient admissions, transfers, and escalation of care to ensure roles and responsibilities are clear under the collaborative telehealth arrangement. If the telehealth consulting provider is not documenting in the patient originating site's local EHR, there needs to be an alternative process to ensure clinical documentation is incorporated in the legal medical record. The agreed financial arrangements would also inform documentation for professional billing and/or contractual payments (e.g. "pay per click" payment models). If the patient originating site is the patient's home, special considerations are made for the patient's device, connectivity, and digital literacy, and an emergency protocol is developed to establish a plan of escalation in case the patient's status declines and additional support is needed.

9.3.3 Emergency plans and procedures

Incidents that disrupt the normal delivery of a telehealth service are bound to occur, and it is essential that the clinical and technical teams are knowledgeable of, and trained on, all documented emergency procedures. A technical incident may be as simple as a bad video connection or as complex as a natural disaster (e.g. a hurricane) that causes an internet outage in a region. Telehealth teams create emergency plans during Development and provide training on those plans during Implementation. A simple approach to telehealth emergency plans is to consider what would occur prior to having the telehealth service, which may include a provider-to-provider telephone call or patient transfer.

Patient safety emergency plans are also created in case a patient needs rapid escalated care. One example is where a provider is conducting a telepsychiatry session, and the patient indicates they are suicidal during the session. Patient safety emergency plans are reviewed thoroughly with any collaborating partners. When care is being delivered directly into a patient's home, emergency plans include having the provider confirm the patient's location at the beginning of the telehealth session in case emergency services may need to be called.

9.3.4 Scheduling protocol

Scheduling protocols are created and reviewed with the respective scheduling offices and relevant providers. The scheduling approach will differ depending on the type of service delivered. Some examples are an around-the-clock (24/7) emergency consultative service (e.g. telestroke), a service that conducts consultations during routine business hours (e.g. ambulatory care), or a service offering continuous remote monitoring (e.g. tele-ICU). For planned telehealth interactions particularly, scheduling considerations apply to patients and clinical staff at the originating site to ensure the right patient sees the right provider at the right time with the necessary ancillary clinical information.

Appropriate scheduling will increase provider and patient engagement in telehealth through efficient and effective use of time. In addition to logistics, scheduling protocols need to address which patient conditions are and are not appropriate for telehealth visits (e.g. chronic condition management vs. acute exacerbation), the telehealth modality (e.g. video visit), and whether the provider is accepting new patients or only previously established patients.

9.3.5 Training protocol

A training protocol outlines who will be trained, how they will be trained, and what information and training will be provided. As a component of the training protocol, supporting documents and/or videos can be created to help educate the providers and supporting care team members on the new workflow and systems. A tip sheet document with screenshots of key features of the telehealth platform and/or EHR can provide the care team members with a visual depiction of the process to initially review, and can assist during the early stages of Implementation.

Similar education and training materials are created for the patient originating site (e.g. hospital, clinic). The training materials include an overview of the telehealth equipment and platform functionality, such as how to request a telehealth encounter and how to use the peripheral devices. In addition, it is beneficial to provide the patient originating site staff with applicable clinical decision criteria on how to select a patient who is appropriate for the telehealth service. Finally, documents and training are provided to the clinical staff at the patient originating site on how to "telepresent" a patient for the consulting provider. This process differs according to specialty, but at a minimum, the telepresenter can use the SBAR technique (Situation, Background, Assessment, Recommendation) and give the consulting provider any relevant medical information (e.g. medication, allergies, medical history, chief complaint) required to make an assessment, and support the consulting provider with any hands-on needs (e.g. gathering vitals, placement of electronic stethoscope, use of examination camera).

9.4 Technology pathway

In Development, a technology needs assessment is conducted to identify what hardware devices will be needed at both the internal (consulting provider) and external (patient) locations. Hardware devices are procured, configured, and deployed as needed to support the service, and a technical support plan is created to ensure personnel are available to respond to incidents. In addition, technology system changes and integrations are completed to support the clinical workflow. Finally, site-to-site technology testing is conducted to confirm that the equipment is working as intended and that adequate connectivity is available to deliver the service successfully.

9.4.1 Technology needs assessment

A formalized technology needs assessment is conducted in the beginning of Development. This process assesses both internal and external technology needs, including hardware devices and connectivity evaluation. The hardware devices required internally may be for the providers delivering the service. External hardware devices are evaluated for compatibility with the telehealth software solution and adequate connectivity to receive the telehealth service. Any new technology needs are fulfilled using existing procurement processes.

9.4.2 Technical support plan

As new telehealth services are created, a technical support plan is established to guarantee that the users of the service (e.g. providers, patients) have a resource to call when technical incidents occur. Ideally, this plan is integrated into existing help desk infrastructure. One of the challenges is that traditional help desk operations have been established to support internal care team members and are not available to patients or external (collaborating) partner sites. Many telehealth platform companies also offer technical support for their solutions. Local decisions will need to be made on how the technical support plan will function, what resources will be allocated to support the service, and which customers it will serve.

9.4.3 Technology system changes and integrations

Once the clinical workflow is reviewed and finalized, the clinical pathway intersects with the technology pathway, and system changes and integrations may be necessary. System changes may be simple configurations within an EHR or granting access to new users of a telehealth platform, or conversely they may require significant development (i.e. new build) within the EHR. Integrations between the telehealth platform and the EHR can be beneficial to the delivery of the service, but it is recommended to keep the integrations simple and optimize the workflow through the Continuous Quality Improvement phase. Understanding the impact of technology system changes and integrations will assist with providing the clinical champions and other relevant stakeholders a realistic time frame for the development of the service. If system changes or integrations are required, test scripts are created to validate that the changes resulted in the intended outcome. The testing of the system changes and integrations is completed within the Development phase.

9.4.4 Technology testing

After the technology hardware devices (e.g. telehealth carts, laptops) are deployed and installed, testing is conducted between the patient originating site and the consulting provider's endpoints. Ensuring the telehealth technology functions appropriately before Implementation will help avoid go-live delays and frustration with clinical champions. It is recommended to conduct standard test scripts to confirm the basic function of the telehealth technology. During this testing, connectivity is also evaluated to ensure that adequate internet speed and bandwidth is available to support the successful delivery of the telehealth service.

9.5 Legal and regulatory pathway

In Development, telehealth teams use the legal and regulatory pathway to confirm that the clinical workflow is compliant with all state and federal regulations, the providers are authorized to deliver the services, and any required legal documentation has been executed or completed prior to go-live (see Figure 9.3). Legal counsel and compliance personnel are consulted on the service-specific clinical workflow to confirm that all applicable regulatory elements (e.g. informed consent, billing documentation) are accounted for and approved. Tasks are completed to ensure that the providers have the appropriate licensure, malpractice coverage, privileging, and credentialing to deliver the telehealth service. Finally, if the telehealth service is being delivered within a partner site (e.g. hospital, school), telehealth agreements must be drafted, negotiated, and executed to detail each party's legal obligations, including any associated compensation.

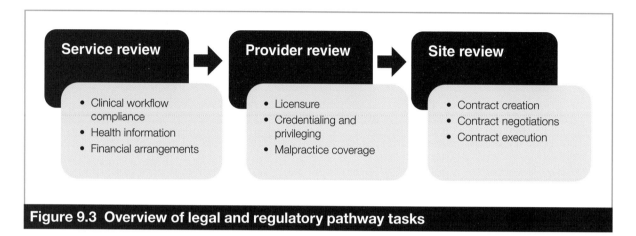

Figure 9.3 Overview of legal and regulatory pathway tasks

9.5.1 Legal and regulatory – service review

The legal and regulatory service review occurs simultaneously with the clinical workflow creation, so that the associated processes and financial arrangements can be reviewed and approved by legal and compliance experts. Examples of service-specific tasks include reviewing patient informed consent requirements and ensuring documentation and billing is compliant with regulatory policies. The exchange of health information within the telehealth service is also scrutinized in order to secure the protection of health information (e.g. HIPAA). Financial arrangements are analyzed to assess whether the pricing of the telehealth service and any related compensation to the consulting providers is fair market value and compliant with state and federal regulations.

9.5.2 Legal and regulatory – provider review

The first legal and regulatory provider task is to confirm that the telehealth service providers are licensed to deliver care in that state. Next, the providers must be credentialed and privileged to deliver the service by their own organization and by any partnering organization that requires credentialing within its bylaws (e.g. a hospital). If applicable, tasks are completed to ensure the providers can legally perform the services and have appropriate approvals from associated hospital medical boards. Finally, a review of the provider's malpractice insurance plan is conducted to confirm coverage of the new telehealth service.

9.5.3 Legal and regulatory – site review

When a partner site is receiving the telehealth service, an agreement is created to outline the terms of the arrangement. The telehealth agreement should clearly document the mutually agreed legal arrangement, the associated obligations of the service, and compliance with all applicable rules and regulations. As healthcare organizations begin to scale their telehealth services, it is beneficial to develop templated agreements for different services when external partnerships are involved. The contract will define the financial arrangement, the length of the partnership, and any language that would allow for the agreement to be terminated. The contractual process can be lengthy as final terms are negotiated and the final agreement is executed. The legal process to execute an agreement should be factored into any go-live timeline projections.

9.6 Outcomes pathway

During the Development phase, the telehealth metrics identified in Strategy are built into data reports for operational monitoring. Standardized telehealth metrics to assess operational performance include utilization, provider experience, patient experience, quality of care delivery, technical reliability, and sustainability. Data sources are identified for each metric, and the data collection process is finalized. Finally, the data reports are validated through testing. The data reports are then scheduled to be delivered at a set cadence for respective decision-makers. Telehealth administrative leaders and clinical champions monitor daily and/or weekly reports to oversee the adoption and operations of the service. Executive leaders receive monthly and/or quarterly reports for more strategic guidance.

9.7 Launch status brief

The launch status brief (LSB) is the final step in the Development phase and is considered the final review of all of the applicable Development tasks. The LSB is a detailed review and final sign-off of the technical and operational requirements and the readiness of the team. During this step, once all of the Development tasks have been confirmed as completed, a projected go-live date is set, and the service advances into the Implementation phase. It should be noted that the LSB meetings may be recurring over a period of time at the end of the Development phase, as an opportunity to bring the project team together to help finalize the remaining tasks.

In addition, an executive decision could be made to advance a service into the Implementation phase with one or more remaining Development tasks. This decision would result in the LSB meetings carrying over into the Implementation phase. It is recommended to permit this only if the remaining Development tasks are imminently pending and will not negatively impact the initial education and training tasks within Implementation. Examples of common scenarios when LSB meetings would continue into Implementation include where the telehealth contract is being signed but not executed yet, or credentialing is not completed but is expected prior to the go-live. It is important to note that the service cannot go live until all of the Development tasks have been completed.

10 | TSIM phase: Implementation

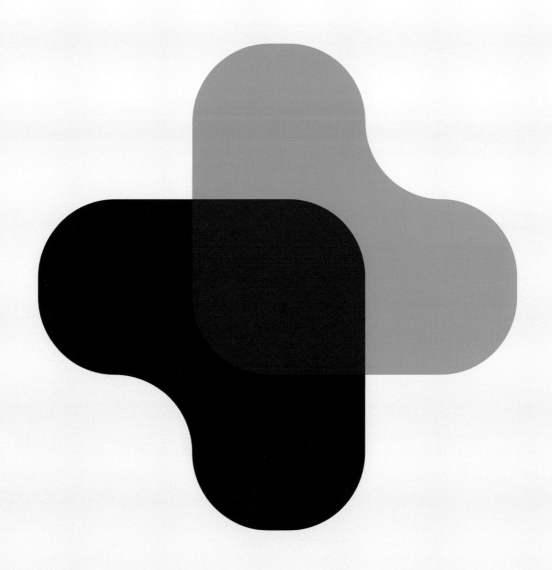

10.1 Introduction

The Implementation phase is when the training, testing, and telehealth service go-live occur. Clinical providers and supporting clinical teams are trained on both the telehealth technology and clinical workflows, and how these integrate into their existing clinical care duties. Technical training for clinicians includes the use of telehealth equipment, mock calls to test workflows, and completion of a successful visit. Service launch dates are established for full program activation. Meticulous communication and significant technical and operational support are imperative, as clinician frustration and discouragement during the Implementation phase will have a significant long-term impact on provider engagement and may threaten program success. Change management is a core process principle that is essential to the successful completion of the activities within the Implementation phase, including the implementation roundtable, training and mock calls, a pre-go-live brief, go-live, and a post-go-live debrief (see Figure 10.1).

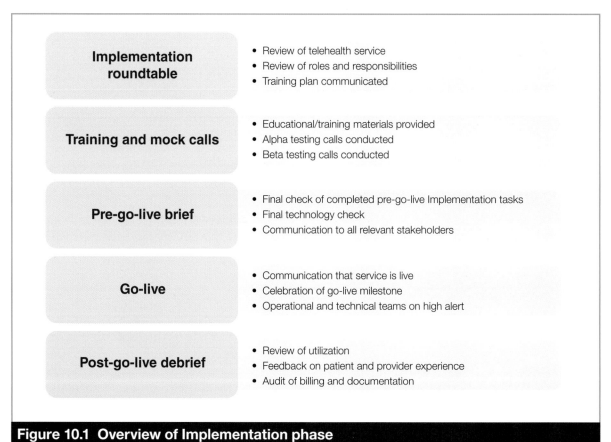

Figure 10.1 Overview of Implementation phase

10.2 Change management

Change management is a core process principle of the Implementation phase as formal steps are taken to prepare resources, coordinate personnel, and execute decisions to take the new telehealth service live. New telehealth services will disrupt the traditional delivery system, and challenges are to be expected. These challenges can be navigated with change management strategies such as the use of a clinical champion, ample training provision, and putting technical support teams on high alert. Finally, transparent communication and convening of stakeholders for collective assessment is paramount, to avoid disruption of the service and to maintain provider and clinical team engagement.

10.3 Implementation roundtable

During the implementation roundtable, the internal service providers and support staff review the clinical workflow and training materials that were created in Development. Team members learn their respective roles and responsibilities to properly execute the service, and learn how this new service offering will fit into existing clinical workflows and scheduling processes.

When the service is being delivered to a partnering site, a second implementation roundtable is conducted to review the service with the collaborating (external) team members at the patient originating site. An implementation charter is reviewed and signed off, so expectations are clear on the training provided and the partner site's involvement. The training materials are integrated into the partnering site's clinical education resources and, using a "train the trainer" methodology when possible, extended to new employees as they are onboarded locally. Training resources are reviewed at least annually and updated with any substantial service modification in a timely manner.

10.4 Training and mock calls

Training and mock calls include the collective activities that ensure the clinical providers and their teams receive adequate training and can demonstrate sufficient competency in their duties in order to conduct successful telehealth encounters. The main goal of training is to prepare providers, nurses, and support staff to effectively deliver the telehealth service as designed, document the encounter, and bill appropriately for the service. Internal and external providers, including telepresenters, receive standardized training on the workflow, technologies, emergency plans, and any documentation requirements, and are given the help desk number to call for any incidents.

A telehealth service is first internally tested through mock calls at the site that will be providing the service, designated as alpha testing. After success has been demonstrated in alpha testing, mock calls with the site receiving the telehealth service are conducted. This activity is designated as beta testing, and is also an opportunity for direct training of the referring providers and their teams. This activity allows the clinical teams to independently conduct a mock visit using the workflow planned for when the service is live. Real-time training reiteration is offered, and any questions that arise during the mock call are investigated and answered. Multiple rounds of beta testing mock calls are completed until the telehealth teams delivering and supporting the service demonstrate competency with the workflow.

It is worth noting that direct-to-consumer (DTC) telehealth services also work thorough alpha and beta testing. Beta testing for DTC services includes using a test patient to analyze go-live readiness. Providers and support staff are also given high-level troubleshooting instruction so that they can assist patients, staff, and receiving providers with the initial incident response, when possible, before engaging technology support teams.

Competency assessment is critical. Evaluation metrics (e.g. successful completion of a mock visit under direct supervision) are used to determine whether additional training is required and, ultimately, whether go-live must be delayed until remediation can be offered. Standardized tools such as competency quizzes that assess knowledge of key workflow components can be leveraged to verify and document the competency of large clinical teams. If scheduling is required for the service, great care is taken to ensure that scheduling workflows are understood and demonstrated by all involved schedulers prior to go-live. Scheduling errors can lead to significant dissatisfaction, and should be avoided through comprehensive training and support early in the go-live period. Auditing of scheduling processes and outputs will be assessed in the post-go-live debrief after a predetermined number of telehealth encounters have been completed.

10.5 Pre-go-live brief

The pre-go-live brief is the final touchpoint of formal communication prior to go-live. This forum is used to confirm the go-live date and time. It also serves to ensure all stakeholders understand their respective roles and responsibilities before, during, and immediately following go-live. A checklist can be used to confirm and communicate responsibilities during the pre-go-live brief to verify readiness.

Here is an example of a pre-go-live brief checklist:

- **Provider equipment readiness** Equipment at provider's location of care (clinic, office, home, etc.) is checked for connectivity as part of technology setup
- **EHR access** EHR accounts applied for, verified, and tested by provider; training offered and support mechanisms outlined
- **Billing plan and routing build** Billing plan is aligned with contractual obligations, internal and external regulations, and compliance, and routed to intended revenue cycle portal
- **Training materials complete and disseminated** Enduring educational materials, tip sheets, emergency plans, and help desk support number shared with all clinical stakeholders
- **Mock calls** Alpha and beta testing calls successfully completed; workflow and technology competency documented
- **Go-live** Date and time confirmed and communicated to all relevant parties

It is important to effectively disseminate the "all clear" for go-live with a summary of the pre-go-live brief through a variety of channels (e.g. meetings, electronic communications). This communication serves as a last call for concerns or requests for additional support from providers and clinical teams, and from technical support teams. In the absence of concerns from stakeholders, the service is on track to go live at the pre-specified date and time.

The pre-go-live brief is the culmination of the extensive work in creating and vetting the development of a service to this point. It is an opportunity to both celebrate and closely manage important details. If even one or two of the pre-go-live brief elements are missing, the implementation will be negatively impacted. Visibility and engagement of administrative telehealth leadership and clinical champions are critical at this point. As telehealth teams acquire experience around these processes, the ability to determine instinctively the readiness of a service or provider group is layered on top of the formal pre-go-live brief. In telehealth, this additional gestalt is representative of a transition along the novice-to-expert continuum for utilization of TSIM.

10.6 Go-live

The go-live is the official implementation of the telehealth service, as defined by offering its availability to patients and/or referring providers. Services vary in their immediate uptake, with some seeing activity on day one and others requiring days or weeks and subsequent awareness campaigns to achieve the first visit. Regardless of immediate service activity, operational and technical support must remain vigilant and on high alert, prepared to respond to any need of the providers, clinical sites, or patients. Stakeholder expectations about go-lives are often difficult to manage, as there are typically varying levels of care team experience with telehealth service go-lives, and normally different levels of technical savvy. Clinical champions and clinical care team members typically do not expect all components of a telehealth service go-live to work perfectly on day one. However, they rightly expect that both operational and technical support teams will respond quickly when issues arise. The initial go-live time period can be crucial to long-term telehealth adoption for providers, and early failures that are not quickly recovered can push providers away from telehealth towards the default and familiar in-person workflows. Real-time support in anticipation of early incidents, even if none occur, is effort well spent in the long run. Similarly, downtime workflows prepared in advance for potential use will pay dividends if and when a backup plan needs to be initiated.

On the day of go-live, it is critical that all stakeholders have been prepared via education, training, and mock calls, and that support resources are readily available. Mission-critical preferences of providers and sites should be respected, and relevant resources should be integrated into existing processes for ease of use. For example, if a provider prefers electronic tip sheets saved on the desktop to paper tip sheets, these preferences should be accommodated to make the provider comfortable.

It is common for the initial telehealth visits to require significant support, and to yield follow-up questions for clarification. This dialogue is critical to hardwiring workflows and related processes. Time allocated to significant support during the go-live period, even when the workflow seems to be running smoothly, can be a differentiator in provider and care team engagement, and enables successful completion of the encounters and accurate documentation. The difference between a mock call and a real patient telehealth visit should not be underestimated, as challenges often develop in the real encounter setting that are not present in the mock call (e.g. digital literacy, EHR navigation challenges, and peripheral operation). Regardless of preparation, inevitable challenges will arise that require support, but these incidents can be quickly resolved with the support of a team ready to troubleshoot in real time. The Implementation phase of hypervigilant support varies in length according to service complexity, provider experience and learning curve, and patient population served.

10.7 Post-go-live debrief

It is important that telehealth teams do not view go-live as the conclusion of the telehealth service development activities. If multiple telehealth services are being developed concurrently, a common pitfall of the telehealth team is to shift from the just-launched service to a new service under development. Disciplined focus on the service in the post-go-live period will offer time to reflect on successes and opportunities for improvement, provide for structured analysis of lagging service success indicators (e.g. billing revenue, documentation compliance), and hardwire services for sustained success.

Typically, a debrief is scheduled following service go-live and after a steady volume of telehealth interactions has been reached over a predetermined period. The requisite volume and time frames will vary according to service type and demand. For example, a telestroke service at a bustling emergency department will likely have enough volume and experience to substantiate a debrief within several weeks, while a small primary care support service offering nutrition counseling may take months to achieve adequate volume before a formal review can inform opportunities for improvement. Regardless of timing and telehealth interaction volumes, carefully tracking the service for a formal post-go-live debrief is important for assessing quality, reliability, and sustainability. It is not uncommon to see organic workflow modifications and billing shortcuts that evolve between go-live and the post-go-live debrief audit. Typically, these unanticipated or unwarranted changes in process will require additional education and training or formal workflow modification, along with documentation or EHR routing optimizations.

Prior to the post-go-live debrief, patient and provider experience are surveyed to assess satisfaction with the delivery of the service, and documentation and billing is audited to ensure compliance with the original design. At the post-go-live debrief, the feedback and audits are reviewed and opportunities for improvement are identified. Providers and clinical staff are offered additional training, if necessary, and small improvements are implemented using a structured continuous quality improvement process.

During the post-go-live debrief, several considerations and outcome metrics are reviewed in detail (see example below). The overarching question in a post-go-live debrief is "Did the service achieve the desired results?" The success metrics identified during Strategy are reviewed. It is common for findings to be preliminary during the debrief; however, it is still relevant to review them for awareness and focus. The results should be communicated to key stakeholders, and a service should not advance into the Operations phase unless all the elements in the post-go-live debrief have demonstrated success. If additional provider training or service education is required, it is conducted, and another ("secondary") debrief is scheduled in the future to reassess the service. Furthermore, a service is deemed appropriate for Operations when volume and success metrics warrant confidence that the intense support offered in the Implementation phase can be relaxed and operational efficiency monitoring can begin.

Here is an example of a post-go-live debrief review list:

- **Utilization data** Are telehealth referring and consulting providers/teams requesting and using the service as expected? Is the service demand as expected? Are there awareness improvement opportunities / marketing resources available?

- **Documentation and billing audit** Are the providers documenting correctly per compliance guidance? Are the providers consistently using the correct billing codes? Are those codes being processed correctly through the system and sent to the payors? Are the payors reimbursing as expected?

- **Patient and provider experience** What is the feedback from the patients receiving care? What is the feedback from the partner site (providers and care team)? What is the feedback from the service providers and care teams? Could the workflow be more efficient? Could the technical reliability be improved? Are there themes in feedback that can be addressed immediately?

- **Service success** How will success be sustained? How will risks be mitigated? What are the provider, patient, or site educational needs at this time? How can the service's successes to date be recognized?

- **Operations phase entry** Is the service ready to move into the Operations phase for sustained operational efficiency support?

11 | TSIM phase: Operations

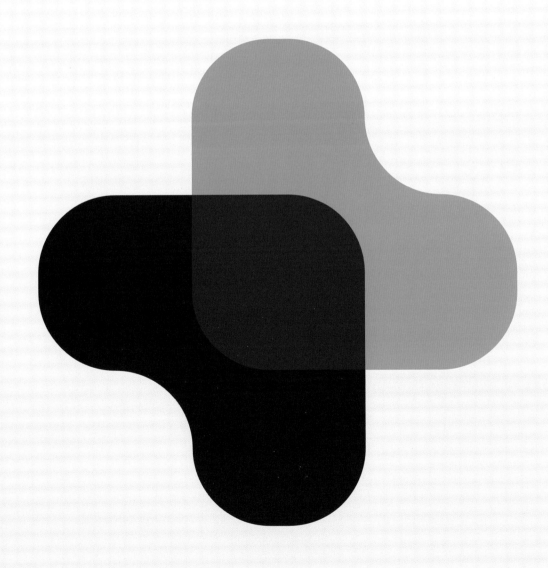

11.1 Introduction

Operations is the culmination of the extensive work done in the Strategy, Development and Implementation phases. Once a telehealth service reaches this phase, alignment between strategic planning and the operational reality is evaluated from multiple stakeholder perspectives. The primary goal in the Operations phase is to deliver highly reliable, high-quality telehealth services that continue to improve quality of care and the patient and provider experience. In this phase, the operational team works to support the increased adoption of the telehealth service and to help it meet the needs of the customers (e.g. partnering hospital sites, patients).

In order to coordinate and direct operational efficiency, telehealth administrative leadership manages a set of two standard operational domains: service delivery management and operational technology management. These both have specific components that can serve as a foundation for creating standard operating procedures (SOPs) to evolve as the telehealth service matures (see Figure 11.1).

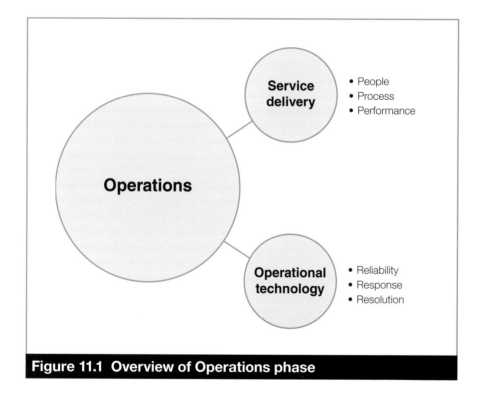

Figure 11.1 Overview of Operations phase

11.2 Service delivery management

Service delivery management is the first domain of the Operations phase. It can be described at a high level as the management of day-to-day operations to deliver high-quality telehealth services and conduct the supporting functions required to maintain high performance. The service delivery domain includes the operational components of people, process, and performance (see Figure 11.2). The people component includes the functions to ensure customer success and workforce optimization. The process component provides an avenue to confirm compliance and proficiency with established procedures. Performance management ensures that the metrics identified in Strategy are consistently monitored and reported in Operations, and any identified deficits in performance are addressed through Continuous Quality Improvement.

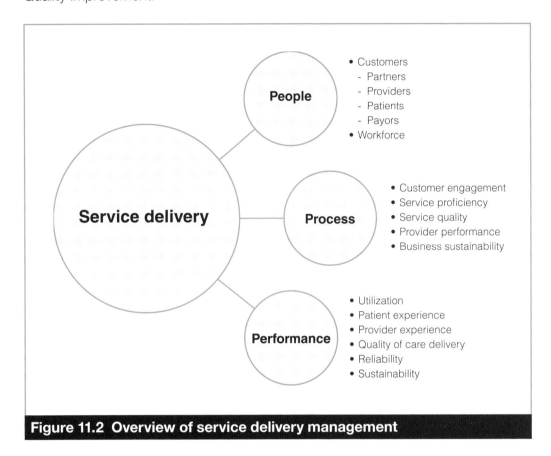

Figure 11.2 Overview of service delivery management

11.2.1 Service delivery – people

The people component focuses on the relationships, perspectives, and success of key "customers" and accounts for the performance of the telehealth team as a whole. The customers can be broken down into four sub-populations: partners, providers, patients, and payors. In addition to customers, operational leadership must effectively manage the workforce delivering and supporting the telehealth services.

The partners of a telehealth service are the people at the collaborating organization who are procuring the telehealth service for patients at their facility. In this example, the executive leadership (e.g. CEO, CMO, CFO) expect to find unique and specific value in the telehealth offering, positively impacting their interests within hospital leadership. Decreasing healthcare costs, improving safety and quality, increasing operational efficiency, and expanding access to care are all examples of how telehealth services can drive value. Recognizing how the value driver related to each telehealth service impacts each partner stakeholder up front will help telehealth leadership manage partner expectations and deliver on value perceptions.

Providers (e.g. physicians) and their supporting care teams, both those who receive and deliver the service, are also customers. Providers who are receiving telehealth services will be interested in service access and efficiency, as well as clinical quality for their patients. It is within their environment (i.e. the patient originating site) that the telehealth service will be delivered, and in order to drive adoption, the telehealth service must be user-friendly and create a perceived value to those physicians and care team members. Providers who are delivering the telehealth service (i.e. the consulting providers) are also customers, and it is essential that their telehealth experience is also perceived as efficient and user-friendly. Like providers at the collaborating organization, the consulting providers want to ensure that the service is delivering high-quality care.

Patients are an additional customer base that could receive the telehealth service within a hospital, a clinic or their home. Patients define value largely by access, efficiency, customer service, and clinical quality. In the hospital setting, they may not have transparent access to value scorecards shared with providers and executive leaders; however, these stakeholders' perceptions of the telehealth service as it relates to their patient experience will drive their healthcare choices and, thus, provider and leader decisions about sustaining telehealth partnerships. When patients are accessing the telehealth services directly (i.e. a direct-to-consumer model), they often expect quality and seek out cost-effective, convenient services.

The third-party payors of telehealth services are also customers. Payors must perceive value in order for them to create favorable reimbursement policies that support the adoption and growth of telehealth services. Payors often perceive value through improvements made in cost-effective care, which can be challenging for telehealth services delivered in a fee-for-service model. As reimbursement models continue to shift towards value-based payment models, the barriers to payment are expected to decline. It is important to maintain good relationships with payors to understand their challenges and provide them with data that informs their policy-making decisions.

Finally, within the people component, there is a workforce management element to ensure team members are fulfilling their roles and responsibilities in order to deliver high-quality telehealth services. The personnel may provide direct clinical care, or they may have a supporting role that directly (e.g. scheduling) or indirectly (e.g. accounts receivable) contributes to the success and sustainability of the service. In addition, there are workforce labor costs that must be managed to ensure the cost relative to the productivity is meeting budgeted expectations and moving towards a successful and sustainable telehealth service.

11.2.2 Service delivery – process

The process component ensures that policies and procedures are hardwired to successfully deliver and sustain telehealth services. Key activities include customer engagement, service proficiency, service quality, provider performance, and business sustainability. The process that supports the people component is customer engagement, which telehealth teams maintain to ensure the service is meeting customers' expectations. Customer engagement is defined as the collective activities used to ensure effective two-way communication and accountability to build trust and maintain a successful telehealth partnership.

Service proficiency is the activity of monitoring and certifying internal and external providers and teams, to ensure they remain sufficiently trained and proficient in the workflow and technology to maintain the successful delivery of the service. Training is an essential activity in the Implementation phase, and should be extended beyond that phase in order to ensure continued proficiency. Ongoing training helps mitigate natural workflow modification challenges that occur related to staff turnover and the process creep associated with human behaviors (e.g. the propensity to take shortcuts to save time). A shared training management relationship between the telehealth team and the partner site is more likely to yield prolonged competency, and to identify education and training needs more readily, as service operations continue from months to years.

Service quality activities identify and address opportunities for improving the delivery of the service. Service quality can be proactively monitored through the data reporting of standardized telehealth metrics in order to assess service improvement opportunities, address educational and training gaps, and resolve quality deficits. Regular report dissemination alone is not sufficient. The service quality reporting process requires multidisciplinary discussion and opportunity for identifying improvements. Benchmarking data is a key driver to goal setting, when available. Shared expectations about service quality metrics, partnership performance, and "highest priority" improvement initiatives are paramount.

The performance of telehealth providers is evaluated at regular intervals to demonstrate and document individual provider proficiency and quality. Ongoing Professional Practice Evaluation (OPPE), a Joint Commission standard, is used in healthcare as a means to evaluate the professional performance of providers to ensure the competency of individual practitioners.[53] As telehealth expands in depth and breadth of service offerings and becomes a more common way of delivering care, organizations and particularly telehealth service customers have begun to request OPPE for telehealth to assess provider proficiency and quality.

Telehealth OPPE can replicate the processes used for in-person care. The domains of evaluation are the same as for in-person care; they include patient care, medical knowledge, systems-based practice, practice-based learning and improvement, and professionalism. Because telehealth experience requires repetition, volume and acuity metrics can be added to the evaluation process. Providers must have a predetermined minimum regular volume to be evaluated for telehealth OPPE and remain privileged.

Telehealth provider evaluations occur every six months, and include a service medical director audit of at least five telehealth encounters for each provider for each service provided. Scoring is filed as part of the provider's general evaluation in the medical affairs office. Feedback from each review is shared by the medical director to the individual providers and additional training or education is offered, as necessary. Remediation is offered where required, based on a score obtained using the standard guidelines issued by The Joint Commission for Focused Professional Practice Evaluation (FPPE). OPPE status reports are shared with partner sites upon request and are reported by service in aggregate. Individual concerns about professional practice from partner sites are shared with telehealth administrative leadership and handled individually. Complaints that are relevant to the OPPE process are filed for integration into the next evaluation period.

Finally, business sustainability includes the comprehensive activities required to maintain the effective operations and ongoing success of the telehealth team. Examples of these business functions may include managing human resources, conducting financial transactions, meeting legal requirements, procuring essential resources to support operations, and marketing key telehealth services. The management of human resources includes, but is not limited to, hiring, training, scheduling staff, and completing payroll. The financial transactions of a telehealth team in Operations may include making payments to telehealth vendors (i.e. accounts payable) and collecting payments on delivered telehealth services (i.e. accounts receivable). As agreements are executed in Development, contractual obligations must be monitored and fulfilled in Operations. Telehealth administrative leadership must identify the resources needed to support the operations of the telehealth services, work with vendors to procure the resources, and track purchases through institutional procurement systems. Finally, ongoing marketing to promote and educate potential customers about the value of the services is essential to the adoption and growth of the services.

11.2.3 Service delivery – performance management

Performance management maintains visibility of all of the telehealth service metrics that were identified in Strategy to ensure the service is meeting expected outcomes. It provides a systematic approach to maintaining quality assurance and identifying opportunities for process improvement. When deficits in performance are observed, the operational team can address them through Continuous Quality Improvement initiatives. In order to have a successful performance management system, data integrity and timely reporting are essential. The standardized telehealth metrics to assess performance are utilization, patient experience, provider experience, quality of care delivery, technical reliability, and sustainability.

11.3 Operational technology management

Operational technology management is the second domain of Operations. It can be described as the management of day-to-day operations for the technical infrastructure, telehealth systems, and devices to ensure that services maintain high reliability, and when incidents occur, that there is a team ready to respond and resolve them as soon as possible (see Figure 11.3). Similar to service delivery, this domain has multiple critical partnerships and business-customer relationships: for example, with software and hardware vendors, network infrastructure teams, information security staff, IT (e.g. EHR) personnel, and the end users themselves.

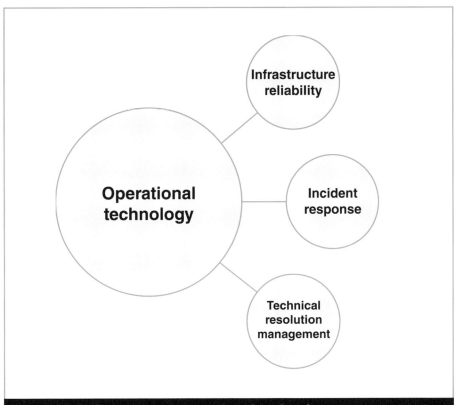

Figure 11.3 Overview of operational technology management

11.3.1 Operational technology – infrastructure reliability

Infrastructure reliability is the process of maintaining a highly reliable telehealth network of hardware and software technologies. Its purpose is to proactively oversee the infrastructure and platforms used by the telehealth team, including those platforms offered by external service providers and telehealth technology vendors. Examples of infrastructure pillars include broadband internet with sufficient bandwidth for transmission of audio and video data, servers to maintain myriad software components and their interoperability, system integrations, software licensing / update management, and information security maintenance.

At a high level, infrastructure reliability maintenance might be described as constant technology "gardening" behind the scenes. This gardening activity is required to maintain the reliability of the telehealth system infrastructure and ultimately avoid catastrophic failures that would impact all stakeholders and disrupt care via interconnected telehealth modalities. Detection of infrastructure failure points is identified via incident monitoring; however, the primary goal of infrastructure reliability maintenance is to *avoid* these failure points and the associated response and resolutions.

11.3.2 Operational technology – incident response

Incident response is the process of quickly identifying and responding to "incidents," defined as any unintended event that adversely impacts the delivery of the telehealth service. Incidents may stem from personnel, process, or technical issues. The telehealth service help desk is the first line of defense to receive calls and address or triage incidents as soon as possible. Optimal telehealth help desks are accessible to consulting and referring provider teams, and to patients in scenarios where a telehealth service is providing direct-to-consumer/patient care.

Incidents are simultaneously tracked through an incident management system to document the incident, including who was involved and, if applicable, its resolution and how long it took to resolve. This system is typically a portal used for service ticket entry. Within the portal, end users have accounts that allow access to the system for real-time ticket entry. Tickets submitted through this portal are reviewed and investigated. Ticket resolution time typically ranges from a few minutes to several days, depending on complexity and compounding factors. Incident response offers data reports that provide an analysis on type of incident, ticket response time (to initiate investigation), and time to ticket resolution. These reports help telehealth teams to better understand their technical reliability and incident response capabilities. In addition to collecting the type of incident, it is beneficial to track and log the engineer's diagnosis and recurrence rate, to better understand infrastructure challenges and the frequency of incidents. Incident response reports are regularly reviewed for trends and opportunities for improvement in technology-related operational efficiency.

11.3.3 Operational technology – technical resolution management

Technical resolution management is the process to manage and create resolutions to identified problems, defined as the accumulation of incidents indicating a larger technical reliability concern with the delivery of telehealth services. Technical resolution is a continuation of incident response, as multiple incident investigations of the same type or cause lead to problem classification. A problem often needs deeper investigation than a simple incident, and typically requires cross-team collaboration. Problems are escalated to telehealth administrative leadership, and if a resolution will take additional time and resources while the service remains impacted, stakeholders and customers are notified. A predetermined process for problem and resolution notification, including scripting, and an update frequency cadence that customers can rely upon is paramount. Email listservs and communication dissemination trees are tactics that can enable timely communication of problems, downtimes, subsequent resolutions, and the return to normal operations. Templated communication components are also helpful. Examples of beneficial communication components in these messages include a description of the situation, the impacted systems and users, a brief description of the action taken to resolve the problem, and the anticipated time to resolution.

12 | TSIM phase: Continuous Quality Improvement

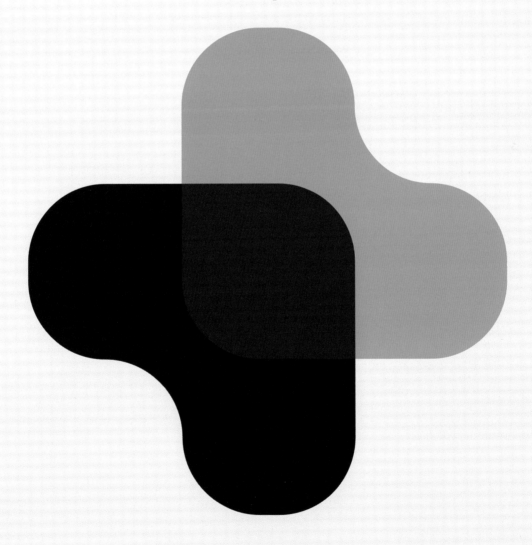

12.1 Introduction

Traditional healthcare systems and processes are notoriously inefficient and have well-documented issues of low quality and value.[54] Telehealth has increasingly been identified as a tool to mitigate problems related to cost, access, and quality. Conversely, there is concern that inserting telehealth into inefficient healthcare systems may merely exacerbate these problems by providing additional opportunities for waste, error, and mismanagement. It is therefore essential that telehealth services have robust quality assurance and improvement processes in place. This is the overarching goal of the Continuous Quality Improvement (CQI) phase of TSIM.

12.2 Challenges of the CQI phase

There are multiple challenges and barriers to the CQI phase that teams should be aware of. These include issues with data collection and monitoring, and failure to maintain standardized evidence-based processes. A recent pitfall of healthcare delivery is an abundance of data, resulting in "data paralysis." The sheer volume of data available in the EHR can make it difficult to interpret the large number of potential outcomes, which may appear to trend in different directions. It is essential to avoid excessive measurement, as the collection and analysis of data can be a resource-intensive endeavor.[55] Measurement strategies should be periodically assessed for usability, utility, and relevance.[56] In addition, the simple act of collecting and sharing performance data does not guarantee improvement.[57] Team members must remember to examine and act on the data.

Another challenge can be a lack of data, as telehealth services often experience significant challenges in obtaining the desired data. This could be due to the difficulties in customizing proprietary vendor platforms for data collection and export. Additionally, telehealth services often require collaboration between separate and independent organizations (i.e. originating and distant sites). Data use agreements may be necessary to ensure the appropriate data is captured and aggregated from both ends of the patient encounter.

Many telehealth services are small, remaining in pilot phases for long periods of time. Therefore, detecting significant clinical, operational, or technical deviations in performance can be challenging, and in rare cases, substantial periods of time can elapse before there is data to examine.[58] Collaboration with health service researchers, informatics specialists, and data analysts can facilitate the appropriate use of data analysis methods, visualization, and interpretation of results. For telehealth services that remain at small volume for a prolonged period, reassessment of the strategy and role to the overall mission should be considered.

A concern with all CQI efforts is that people tend to revert to old habits, or find workarounds and shortcuts to established procedures. It is important that the CQI teams develop maintenance and sustainability procedures in their activities, which can include checklists, incentives, ongoing training, and monitoring. Another component of maintenance consists of tools such as leadership rounds, where telehealth service leaders can observe and monitor front-line care delivery.

12.3 Building high reliability into telehealth services

In the CQI phase, quality improvement methodologies are used to improve processes, which in turn will lead to improved outcomes.[59] During the Strategy and Development phases, planning for service-level metrics, data tracking, monitoring, and evaluation takes place. Throughout the service's maturation, CQI provides a process to allow realigning the telehealth service to meet the evolving needs of patients and providers, and to ensure high reliability. High-reliability organizations (HROs) are organizations that have systems in place to enable consistent achievement of organizational goals. HROs typically experience fewer problems than peer healthcare organizations due to organizational mindfulness and a dominant safety culture[60] (see Table 12.1). The goal of the TSIM CQI phase is to embed the characteristics of an HRO within the telehealth service.

Table 12.1: Characteristics of high reliability

Component	Definition
Preoccupation with failure	All team members are cognizant about the potential for telehealth service failures. New threats and potential problems are acknowledged as situations that can occur regularly. A lack of identified errors could lead to complacency or a false perception of safety. Instead, near misses are viewed as learning opportunities to identify areas that need stronger attention, and to examine possibilities for improvement.
Reluctance to simplify	Team members understand that telehealth services are complex and evolving. Over-simplification of processes or mistakes is risky. It is essential to understand the underlying mechanisms and strive to standardize workflows to reduce variation.
Sensitivity to operations	Teams have a continuous awareness of the systems, processes, and context of the telehealth service. An understanding of the current situations and how they may reinforce or discourage safety is essential.
Deference to expertise	Leaders must be willing to listen to front-line staff, who understand how day-to-day processes are conducted. All team members are expected to report safety concerns or potential problems.
Commitment to resilience	There is an acknowledgement that telehealth services are complex, and failures can occur. Team members must understand the risks of failure and be prepared to identify issues and respond appropriately when issues occur, to mitigate negative or unintended consequences.

(Sources: Weick and Sutcliffe, 2015[61]; Hines et al., 2008[62])

12.4 CQI throughout TSIM

The lens of CQI spans across every phase of TSIM, as opportunities for improvement can be identified both in the project management areas of Development and Implementation and in the service management area of Operations. In Development and Implementation, CQI opportunities typically involve the people, processes, and activities needed to take the telehealth service from Strategy to the post-go-live debrief in Implementation. When a service is in Operations, CQI may be focused on optimizing a process, improving a technology, or educating and training people.

In CQI, key performance indicators (KPIs) are continuously examined by leadership to monitor trends, identify and recommend opportunities for improvement, and maintain the overall value of the telehealth service. KPIs should be updated as close to real time as possible, so that problems or negative trends can be quickly identified. Accurate and timely data is imperative to inform decision-making and enhance program outcomes to meet customers' needs. There are four components of ensuring telehealth services meet the customers' needs: quality planning, quality assurance, quality improvement, and innovation.[63,64,65]

12.4.1 Quality planning

Quality planning takes place during the Strategy and Development phases, where service evaluation plans are created. Identifying standardized success metrics (i.e. KPIs) in Strategy and building a data collection and reporting plan in Development ensures data can be used in a format that facilitates quality improvement and data-driven decision-making. The structure of TSIM guarantees that quality planning occurs early in the process of developing telehealth services.

12.4.2 Quality assurance

Quality assurance, also called "quality control," occurs in Operations, where performance is monitored for deviations between service outcomes and established goals. Telehealth leadership is engaged in the monitoring of service KPIs to ensure customer needs are met and services are meeting established benchmarks. The telehealth team will track metrics in Operations through performance management by monitoring utilization, patient experience, provider experience, quality of care delivery, technical reliability, and financial sustainability. Statistical process control tools, such as run and control charts, and data visualization are used to examine performance.[66] Any KPI that is out of compliance with established benchmarks is assigned to a multidisciplinary process improvement team for further investigation.

12.4.3 Quality improvement

At the core of the CQI phase is quality improvement, where processes are systematically studied and improved. The key areas of CQI are the telehealth services' processes and workflows, the technology, and the training and education needs of the stakeholders. It is important that the CQI team includes members from all levels of the telehealth team, including leadership, which is important for gaining buy-in and support for resource needs. Inclusion of front-line staff is also essential, as they understand the day-to-day delivery of the service and barriers to achieving ideal processes. Other important members include those with clinical expertise and those with technical expertise in quality improvement, change management, project management, training, and data analysis.[67] Depending on the needs of the particular project, ad-hoc CQI working group members with specific expertise may be pulled in to focus on specific topics (e.g. billing and compliance).

12.4.4 Innovation

Finally, in some cases, the team working on CQI will identify that an existing telehealth service can no longer meet the customer's needs, even with extensive process improvement. In this case, innovation is needed to develop new approaches.[68] This could occur for a variety of reasons. For example, a new technology may become available, new regulations may be implemented, or a new customer population may have needs that cannot be met by existing services. Under any of these scenarios, the service will move back to the Strategy phase and either work through the activities again or be discontinued.

In contrast to service optimization, which involves redesigning adjacent services that fit within the existing delivery model, innovation includes designing a new service to meet unmet stakeholder needs.[69] A formalized process is established to submit, review, and prioritize optimization and innovation requests through a committee structure. Innovation requests and ideas will likely need to be vetted through the Pipeline phase and continue through the TSIM framework.

12.5 Service optimization

Unless the strategy of the service is changing, optimization requests do not need to go through the full TSIM framework. The service optimization requests that have been reviewed and prioritized can go through a pre-check meeting to communicate the upcoming change, which could be to modify a process or implement a new technology. At the pre-check meeting, Development tasks that are required to complete the optimization are identified. The completion of these tasks will follow the normal Development approach into Implementation, where new training, mock calls, and a go-live are established for the optimization.

12.6 CQI tools

The CQI phase requires structure, tools, and best practices for improvement. There are well-established models to guide the CQI phase, including Plan-Do-Study-Act (PDSA) cycles, Lean Management, Total Quality Management, and Six Sigma. A common approach is the PDSA cycle. This model uses three foundational questions and the PDSA cycle to guide CQI (see Figure 12.1). Through application of PDSA, CQI teams will create a quality improvement plan to describe the procedures that will be followed to facilitate improvement.

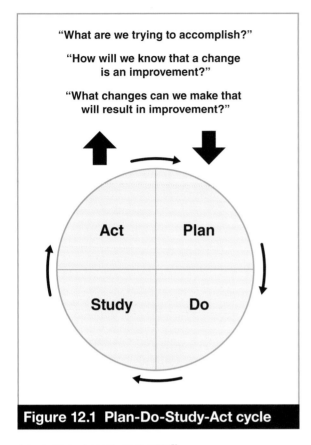

"What are we trying to accomplish?"

"How will we know that a change
is an improvement?"

"What changes can we make that
will result in improvement?"

Act Plan

Study Do

Figure 12.1 Plan-Do-Study-Act cycle

Adapted from Langely *et al.*, 1994[70]

The first question is "What are we trying to accomplish?" The CQI team will identify goals for improvement, also known as aim or goal statements. These statements are written in a "SMART" format, where the goal is Specific, Measurable, Actionable, Realistic, and Timely.[71] The statements guide improvement activities and data collection, and bind the improvement work to a manageable scale to avoid scope creep.

Next, the CQI team explores, "How will we know that a change is an improvement?" This step is designed to understand the background of the problem and the current practices, and to examine data sources and outcomes. This may require additional drilling down of the standardized telehealth metrics, to further stratify data by patient population, provider, time of service, etc. In this stage, process mapping is an effective tool to identify where problems may be occurring in the delivery of the service.

Cause-and-effect relationships are not always obvious when a problem is initially being examined.[72] Therefore formal root cause analysis methods are used to investigate the underlying cause. In a root cause analysis, the collected data and information is systematically assessed to identify factors that contribute to poor outcomes. One common root cause analysis tool is the "fishbone diagram," also known as the "Ishikawa" or "cause-and-effect diagram," where the problem statement (effect) is listed at the far right of the diagram (see Figure 12.2). Next, data-driven and brainstormed causes of the problem are categorized onto branches of the diagram. The branch category names can be customized to fit the specific problem; common categories include examination of people, process, performance, technical reliability, and incident response. The specific causes are then listed on the "spine" of each category. Each potential cause of the problem is investigated, asking "Why does this occur?" Root cause analysis tools allow the CQI team to move beyond quick reactions and focus on actionable items.

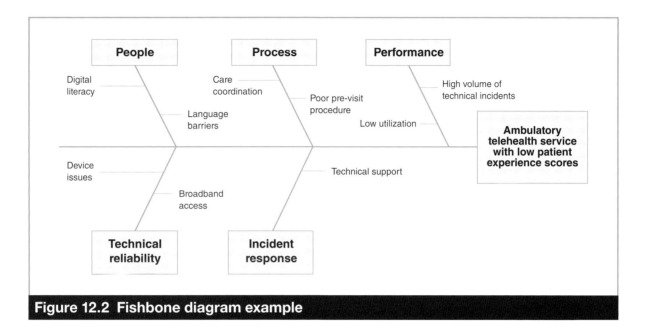

Figure 12.2 Fishbone diagram example

The final question is "What changes can we make that will result in improvement?" After identifying possible changes, the team can prioritize possible improvement approaches. Improvement activities are prioritized based on their ability to impact outcomes, ease of implementation, and cost effectiveness. Tools such as a key driver diagram (see Figure 12.3), which aligns the evidence-based strategies and activities needed to "drive" change and achieve improvement goals, can assist in identifying whether proposed changes are associated with outcomes.[73] For example, a team trying to improve patient experience scores with an ambulatory telehealth service may find key drivers to be related to patients' comfort level with the technology and insufficient technical support provided pre-visit. Change ideas can then focus on evidence-based solutions to enhance the usability and comfort with the technology and process.

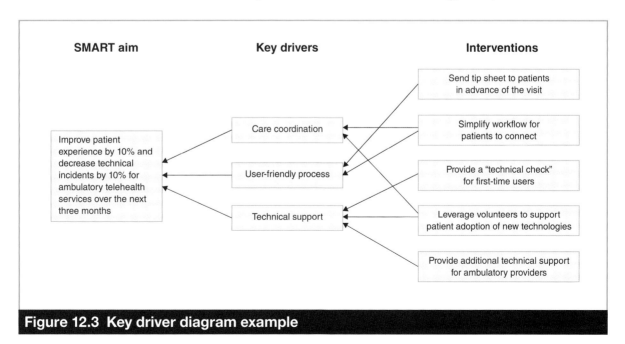

Figure 12.3 Key driver diagram example

After the CQI team has explored these three questions, the PDSA cycle is used to develop, test, and implement changes. Repeated cycles are used to study the impact of small changes to processes, study the results, and respond accordingly. The four components of the PDSA cycle are:

- **Plan** Determine the changes to be implemented and design the improvement plan
- **Do** Implement the changes and document observations
- **Study** Examine the data and results. Under this component, lessons can be learned from both successes and failures
- **Act** Make changes to the process based on the data and lessons learned.

At the conclusion of a single PDSA cycle, the team conducts additional PDSA cycles and implements successful changes into the standard care processes. Early cycles can test the feasibility of changes and examine the impact of changing processes under varying circumstances. Once effective processes are put in place, the CQI team develops a plan to ensure maintenance and sustainability, and continues to monitor the KPIs for quality assurance.

12.7 CQI – efficiency of care

In order to prevent telehealth services adding waste and inefficiencies in the healthcare system, CQI teams should understand the potential areas for waste within the service and strive to eliminate it. There are many types of waste and issues that reduce care quality, including overtreatment, undertreatment, duplication of services, errors, lack of standardization, failure to follow evidence-based practices, lack of care coordination, failures in execution of care processes, administrative complexity, pricing failures, and fraud and abuse.[74,75,76] Specific examples that have already arisen related to telehealth include inappropriate use of antibiotics in direct-to-consumer services, and inefficient implementation of technology.

Often, telehealth services are siloed or small scale. The CQI team should be aware of duplicate efforts and redundant processes, such as different specialty providers remotely monitoring the same patient for different disease states (e.g. diabetes and congestive heart failure). With regard to administrative complexity and potential fraud, a 2018 Office of Inspector General study found that nearly one-third of telehealth claims failed to meet the Medicare billing requirements.[77] Where possible, the telehealth program seeks to maintain economies of scale through centralized resources and standardized processes and technologies.

12.8 Safety culture

There must be a system in place through which stakeholders can submit concerns and safety incidents. This system will include a formal process to conduct quality reviews of incidents, or near misses where an error could have occurred but was identified and stopped prior to initiation. Many healthcare systems have an established mechanism for customer concerns and patient safety reporting. This infrastructure can be expanded and adapted to meet the needs of the telehealth services. Efforts to increase transparency and awareness of the reporting system are necessary to ensure utilization and consistent reporting. A ticketing and routing system sends the information to a telehealth team member for triage. When warranted by the triage evaluation, a multidisciplinary CQI team investigates submissions, using root cause analysis tools and ensuring appropriate follow-up.

It is essential that all stakeholders feel comfortable in identifying and reporting opportunities for improvement, near misses, and safety concerns. To establish these criteria, a safety culture is required.

Components of a safety culture[78] include:

- Recognition of the complex and high-risk nature of the program activities, with an emphasis on maintaining safe operations
- A blame-free environment, where everyone feels safe to report errors and near misses without fear of retribution or retaliation
- Encouragement of interprofessional collaboration to identify and mitigate safety concerns
- Commitment of resources to address safety concerns.

12.9 CQI conclusion

The CQI phase of TSIM is ideally grounded in the principles used by HROs, and involves building a culture of safety and transparency along with supporting the teams with the necessary data and resources to improve outcomes. CQI work begins in the initial phases of TSIM, where teams plan for service outcomes and data collection and, as the name suggests, continues throughout all phases. For optimal CQI, it is essential that telehealth stakeholders feel empowered not only to report errors but also to identify processes that could be standardized and waste that could be eliminated.

13 | TSIM summary

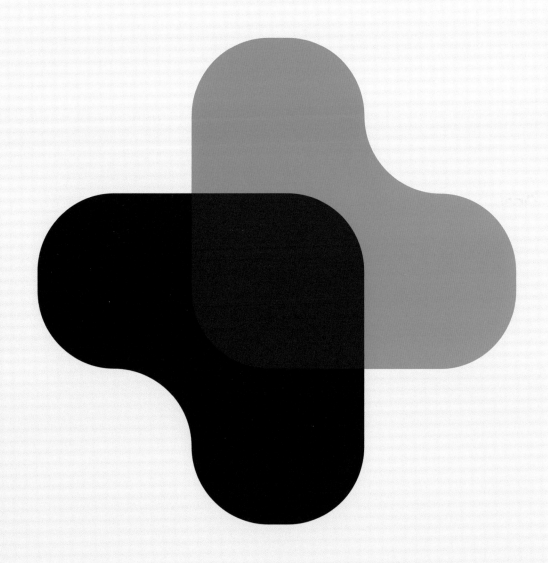

Telehealth has experienced exponential growth over the last decade, and the international COVID-19 pandemic further accelerated this trend as healthcare systems rapidly implemented virtual care delivery solutions. As healthcare organizations attempt to create hybrid care models and integrate telehealth into long-term strategic initiatives, development and implementation challenges are likely to continue without a structured approach guiding and coordinating telehealth teams. The TSIM creators had extensive experience prior to the pandemic in developing, implementing, and operating telehealth services – some successful and some unsuccessful. TSIM is the direct result of this hard-won practical experience in healthcare broadly and telehealth specifically. While it can seem daunting to embark on a telehealth journey, the opportunity to apply innovations to improve quality of care and the patient and provider experience makes the effort well worthwhile.

TSIM offers a structured and practical approach to telehealth service development by breaking down the many processes and steps into logical phases, each grounded and informed by principles of continuous quality improvement. The importance of each phase, and of working through earlier phases prior to moving into later ones, cannot be over-emphasized. Ensuring robust institutional alignment and rigorous focus during Strategy will ultimately enable success during Operations. Covering all processes and steps during Development will ensure clinical, technical, legal, and outcomes planning are rigorously addressed. The careful training and testing during Implementation will ensure the new service is poised for success prior to moving into full Operations. While there is a tendency among novices to want to move directly into Operations, this is a critical error, as it is unlikely to result in a sustainable and scalable telehealth service. TSIM was created to assist and empower healthcare organizations that are embarking on a clinical transformation journey to efficiently and effectively redesign the delivery of healthcare.

Endnotes

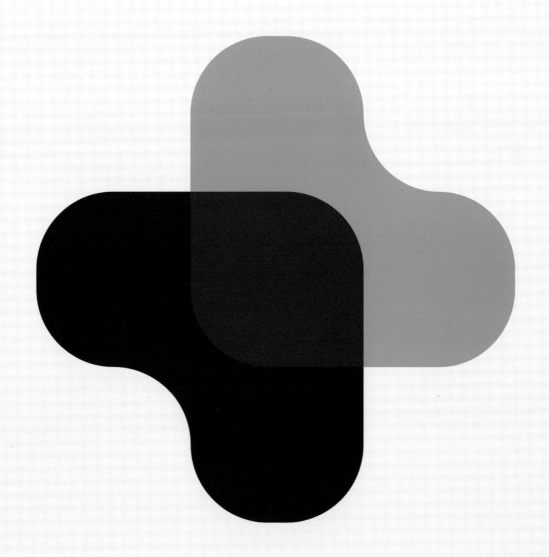

Endnotes

1   US Department of Health & Human Services (2020). Strategic goal 1: Reform, strengthen, and modernize the nation's healthcare system. https://www.hhs.gov/about/strategic-plan/strategic-goal-1/index.html

2   Tikkanen, R. and Abrams, M. (2020). US health care from a global perspective, 2019: Higher spending, worse outcomes? The Commonwealth Fund. https://www.commonwealthfund.org/publications/issue-briefs/2020/jan/us-health-care-global-perspective-2019

3   Health Resources & Services Administration (n.d.). Telehealth programs. https://www.hrsa.gov/rural-health/telehealth

4   Teledoc (2017). Using telehealth to achieve the triple aim. https://www.acoexhibithall.com/wp-content/uploads/2018/02/Using_Telehealth_to_Achieve_the_Triple_Aim_0217.pdf

5   Wang, E. and Day, S. (n.d.). Q3 2020: A new annual record for digital health (already). Rock Health. https://rockhealth.com/reports/q3-2020-digital-health-funding-already-sets-a-new-annual-record/

6   Institute of Medicine (US): Committee on Evaluating Clinical Applications of Telemedicine (1996). Evolution and current applications of telemedicine. In M. J. Field (ed.), *Telemedicine: A Guide to Assessing Telecommunications in Health Care*. National Academies Press (US), Washington, DC. https://www.ncbi.nlm.nih.gov/books/NBK45445/

7   Hunter, T. B. (2014). Teleradiology: A brief overview. The Arizona Telemedicine Program. https://telemedicine.arizona.edu/blog/teleradiology-brief-overview

8   Malykhina, E. (2013). Home is where the health is: Obamacare positions "telehealth" tech as a remedy for chronic hospital readmissions. *Scientific American*. https://www.scientificamerican.com/article/affordable-care-act-technology/

9   Gelburd, R. (2020). Telehealth claims lines increased 4132% nationally from June 2019 to June 2020. *American Journal of Managed Care*. https://www.ajmc.com/view/contributor-telehealth-claim-lines-increased-4132-nationally-from-june-2019-to-june-2020

10 Assistant Secretary for Planning and Evaluation (2020). Medicare beneficiary use of telehealth visits: Early data from the start of the COVID-19 pandemic. https://aspe.hhs.gov/system/files/pdf/263866/hp-issue-brief-medicare-telehealth.pdf

11 Bestsennyy, O., Gilbert, G., Harris, A. and Rost, J. (2020). Telehealth: A quarter-trillion-dollar post-COVID-19 reality? McKinsey & Company. https://www.mckinsey.com/industries/healthcare-systems-and-services/our-insights/telehealth-a-quarter-trillion-dollar-post-covid-19-reality#

12 Verma, S. (2020). Early impact of CMS expansion of Medicare telehealth during COVID-19. Health Affairs blog. https://www.healthaffairs.org/do/10.1377/hblog20200715.454789/full/

13 Mehrotra, A., Linetsky, D. and Hatch, H. (2020). This is supposed to be telemedicine's time to shine. Why are doctors abandoning it? Stat. https://www.statnews.com/2020/06/25/telemedicine-time-to-shine-doctors-abandoning-it/

14 Tanriverdi, H. and Iacono, C. S. (1998). Knowledge barriers to diffusion of telemedicine. In: Proceedings of the International Conference of the Association for Information Systems, Helsinki, Finland, August 14–16. pp 39–50.

15 Lin, C.-C. C., Dievler, A., Robbins, C., Sripipatana, A., Quinn, M. and Nair, S. (2018). Telehealth in health centers: Key adoption factors, barriers, and opportunities. *Health Affairs (Millwood)*. 37: 1967–1974. https://doi.org/10.1377/hlthaff.2018.05125

16 Finch, T. L., Mair, F. S. and May, C. R. (2006). Teledermatology in the UK: Lessons in service innovation. *British Journal of Dermatology*. 156(3): 521–527.

17 Velasquez, D. and Mehrotra, A. (2020). Ensuring the growth of telehealth during COVID-19 does not exacerbate disparities in care. Health Affairs blog. DOI: 10.1377/hblog20200505.591306.

18 Andrus, D. (2020). The future of telehealth is hybrid. BenefitsPRO. https://www.benefitspro.com/2020/10/13/the-future-of-telehealth-is-hybrid/?slreturn=20201127112121

19 Ross, C. (2020). Telehealth grew wildly popular amid Covid-19. Now visits are plunging, forcing providers to recalibrate. Stat. https://www.statnews.com/2020/09/01/telehealth-visits-decline-covid19-hospitals/

20 Wang and Day (n.d.). Q3 2020.

21 MUSC Health (n.d.). A brief history of telehealth at MUSC. https://muschealth.org/medical-services/telehealth/about/history

22 Raths, D. (2019). ATA recognizes telehealth innovators. Healthcare Innovation. https://www.hcinnovationgroup.com/population-health-management/telehealth/news/21076087/ata-recognizes-telehealth-innovators

23 American Association for Respiratory Care (n.d.). How I went from bedside RT to telemedicine. https://www.aarc.org/careers/career-advice/professional-development/how-i-went-from-bedside-rt-to-telemedicine/

24 Van Dyk, L. (2014). A review of telehealth service implementation frameworks. *International Journal of Environmental Research and Public Health*. 11(2): 1279–1298.

25 AXELOS (2019). ITIL – IT service management. AXELOS Global Best Practice. https://www.axelos.com/best-practice-solutions/itil. ITIL® is a registered trade mark of AXELOS Ltd.

26   Hayes, M. (n.d.). MUSC named one of the first National Telehealth Centers of Excellence. https://medicine.musc.edu/departments/dom/annual-report/2018-annual-report/research/telehealth-coe

27   Armstrong, R. L. and Dilley, J. (2021). The consumers guide to internet speed. HighSpeedInternet.com. https://www.highspeedinternet.com/resources/the-consumers-guide-to-internet-speed

28   Pennic, J. (2020). Telehealth and cybersecurity: What you should know. HIT Consultant. https://hitconsultant.net/2020/07/22/telehealth-cybersecurity-what-you-should-know/#.X8Ptps1Kg2w

29   Fruhlinger, J. (2020). What is information security? Definition, principles, and jobs. CSO. https://www.csoonline.com/article/3513899/what-is-information-security-definition-principles-and-jobs.html

30   Mobfilia. (2020). Web API and HL7 FHIR – The future of interoperability. https://www.mobifilia.com/web-api-and-hl7-fhir-the-future-of-interoperability/

31   Center for Connected Health Policy (n.d.). Credentialing and privileging. https://www.telehealthpolicy.us/telehealth-policy/credentialing-and-privileging

32   Legal Information Institute, Cornell Law School (n.d.). Standard of care. https://www.law.cornell.edu/wex/standard_of_care

33   Grady, A. (2005). The importance of standard of care and documentation. *AMA Journal of Ethics*. 7(11): 756–758. https://journalofethics.ama-assn.org/article/importance-standard-care-and-documentation/2005-11

34   American Medical Association (n.d.). Patient-physician relationships. https://www.ama-assn.org/delivering-care/ethics/patient-physician-relationships

35   Center for Connected Health Policy (2021). State telehealth laws and reimbursement policies: Spring 2021. https://cchp.nyc3.digitaloceanspaces.com/2021/04/Spring2021_ExecutiveSummary.pdf

36   Levine, S. J. and Ferrante, T. B. (2020). Telehealth and substance use disorder treatment: Regulatory barriers to entry can mean opportunity for innovative companies. Foley & Lardner LLP.

37   Faget, K., Lacktman, N., Joseph, J. and Shalom, A. (2021). Telehealth legal and regulatory issues. In D. Ford and S. Valenta, *Telemedicine: Overview and Application in Pulmonary, Critical Care, and Sleep Medicine* (pp 15–31). Springer Nature Switzerland AG, Switzerland. https://link.springer.com/book/10.1007/978-3-030-64050-7

38   Hall, J. L. and McGraw, D. (2014). For telehealth to succeed, privacy and security risks must be identified and addressed. *Health Affairs*. 33(2): 216–221. https://doi.org/10.1377/hlthaff.2013.0997

39   HIPAA Journal (n.d.). HIPAA guidelines on telemedicine. https://www.hipaajournal.com/hipaa-guidelines-on-telemedicine/

40   Zhao, M., Hamadi, H., Haley, D. R., Xu, J., White-Williams, C. and Park, S. (2020). Telehealth: Advances in alternative payment models. *Telemedicine and e-Health*. 26(12): 1492–1499. http://doi.org/10.1089/tmj.2019.0294

41   Smeltzer, P., Peterson, T. and Sylvia, M. (2017). Discussion: The value equation in total population health. American Association for Physician Leadership. https://www.physicianleaders.org/news/discussion-the-value-equation-in-total-population-health

42   Zhang, X., Lin, D., Pforsich, H. and Lin, V. W. (2020). Physician workforce in the United States of America: Forecasting nationwide shortages. *Human Resources for Health*. 18(1), article 8. https://doi.org/10.1186/s12960-020-0448-3

43   Worth, T. (2020, October 20). Driving efficiency in virtual care. *Leader's Edge*. https://www.leadersedge.com/healthcare/driving-efficiency-in-virtual-care

44   Adcock, M. and Davis, T. (2018). Remote patient monitoring: A Mississippi success story. Conference session, HIMSS18, Las Vegas, NV. https://365.himss.org/sites/himss365/files/365/handouts/550235296/handout-264.pdf

45   Klein, S. (n.d.). "Hospital at home" programs improve outcomes, lower costs but face resistance from providers and payers. The Commonwealth Fund. https://www.commonwealthfund.org/publications/newsletter-article/hospital-home-programs-improve-outcomes-lower-costs-face-resistance

46   Ford, D., Harvey, J. B., McElligott, J., King, K., Simpson, K. N., Valenta, S., Warr, E. H., Walsh, T., Debenham, E., Teasdale, C., Meystre, S., Obeid, J. S., Metts, C. and Lenert, L. A. (2020). Leveraging health system telehealth and informatics infrastructure to create a continuum of services for COVID-19 screening, testing, and treatment. *Journal of the American Medical Informatics Association*. 27(12): 1871–1877. https://doi.org/10.1093/jamia/ocaa157

47   Davenport, T. and Kalakota, R. (2019). The potential for artificial intelligence in healthcare. *Future Healthcare Journal*. 6(2): 94–98. https://doi.org/10.7861/futurehosp.6-2-94

48   Ibid.

49   National Quality Forum (2017). Creating a framework to support measure development for telehealth. https://www.qualityforum.org/Publications/2017/08/Creating_a_Framework_to_Support_Measure_Development_for_Telehealth.aspx

50   NICE Systems (n.d.). What is Net Promoter? https://www.netpromoter.com/know/

51   Corporate Finance Institute (n.d.). Net profit margin. https://corporatefinanceinstitute.com/resources/knowledge/finance/net-profit-margin-formula/

52   Institute for Healthcare Improvement (n.d.). The IHI Triple Aim. http://www.ihi.org/Engage/Initiatives/TripleAim/Pages/default.aspx

53   The Joint Commission (n.d.). Ongoing professional practice evaluation (OPPE) – Understanding the requirements. https://www.jointcommission.org/standards/standard-faqs/critical-access-hospital/medical-staff-ms/000001500/

54   Berwick, D. M. and Hackbarth, A. D. (2012). Eliminating waste in US healthcare. *Journal of the American Medical Association*. 307(14): 362–365. https://doi.org/10.1001/jama.2012.362

55   Berwick, D. M. (2016). Era 3 for medicine and healthcare. *Journal of the American Medical Association*. 315(13): 1329–1330. https://doi.org/10.1001/jama.2016.1509

56   Quinn Patton, M. (2008). *Utilization-Focused Evaluation*. Fourth Edition. Sage Publications, Saint Paul, MN.

57   Thor, J., Lundberg, J., Ask, J., Olsson, J., Carli, C., Pukk-Harenstam, K. and Brommels, M. (2007). Application of statistical process control in healthcare improvement: Systematic review. *Quality and Safety in Health Care*. 16: 387–399. https://doi.org/10.1136/qshc.2006.022194

58   Ibid.

59   Donabedian A. (1988). The quality of care. How can it be assessed? *Journal of the American Medical Association*. 260(12): 1743–1748. doi: 10.1001/jama.260.12.1743. PMID: 3045356.

60   Weick, K. E. and Sutcliffe, K. M. (2015). *Managing the Unexpected: Sustained Performance in a Complex World*. Third edition. Jossey-Bass, San Francisco, CA. ISBN-13: 9781118862414.

61   Ibid.

62   Hines, S., Luna, K., Lofthus, J. *et al*. (2008). Becoming a high reliability organization: Operational advice for hospital leaders. AHRQ Publication No. 08-0022. Rockville, MD: Agency for Healthcare Research and Quality. https://archive.ahrq.gov/professionals/quality-patient-safety/quality-resources/tools/hroadvice/hroadvice.pdf

63   Bhattacharyya, O., Blumenthal, D., Stoddard, R., Mansell, L., Mossman, K. and Schneider, E. C. (2018). Redesigning care: Adapting new improvement methods to achieve person-centered care. *BMJ Quality & Safety*. 28: 242–248. https://doi.org/10.1136/bmjqs-2018-008208

64   Juran, J. (1989). *Juran on Leadership Quality: An Executive Handbook*. Free Press, New York, NY

65   Recker, D. and Oie, M. (1994). Application of total quality management to unit-based quality assessment and improvement. *Journal of Nursing Care Quality*. 8(4): 25–32. https://doi.org/10.1097/00001786-199407000-00005

66   Thor *et al*. (2007). Application of statistical process control.

67   Knox, L. and Brach, C. (2015). Primary Care Practice Facilitation Curriculum (Module 20). AHRQ Publication No. 15-0060-EF. Agency for Healthcare Research and Quality, Rockville, MD. https://pcmh.ahrq.gov/page/primary-care-practice-facilitation-curriculum

68   Bhattacharyya *et al*. (2018). Redesigning care.

69   Ibid.

70   Langley, G., Nolan, K. and Nolan., T. (1994). The foundation of improvement. *Quality Progress*, June: 81–86.

71   Ogrinc, G. S., Headrick, L.A., Moore, S.M., Barton, A.J., Dolansky, M.A. and Madigosky, W.S. (2012). *Fundamentals of Health Care Improvement: A Guide to Improving Your Patient's Care*. Joint Commission Resources Inc, Institute for Healthcare Improvement. Second edition. Institute for Healthcare Improvement, Cambridge, MA. https://library.uams.edu/assets/fundamentals_of_health_care_improvement.pdf

72   Thor *et al*. (2007). Application of statistical process control.

73   Agency for Healthcare Research and Quality (AHRQ) (2019). Culture of safety. https://psnet.ahrq.gov/primer/culture-safety

74   Bentley, T. G. K., Effros, R. M., Palar, K. and Keeler, E. B. (2008). Waste in the U.S. health care system: A conceptual framework. *The Millbank Quarterly*. 86(4): 629–659.

75   Berwick and Hackbarth (2012). Eliminating waste in US healthcare.

76   Shrank, W. H., Rogstad, T. L. and Parekh, N. (2019). Waste in the US health care system. *Journal of the American Medical Association*. 322(15): 1501–1509. https://doi.org/10.1111/j.1468-0009.2008.00537.x

77   Jarmon, G. L. (2018). CMS paid practitioners for telehealth services that did not meet Medicare requirements. Department of Health and Human Services Office of the Inspector, General Report no. A-05-16-00058. https://oig.hhs.gov/oas/reports/region5/51600058.pdf

78   AHRQ (2019). Culture of safety.

Appendix
Ohio River Health System and TSIM

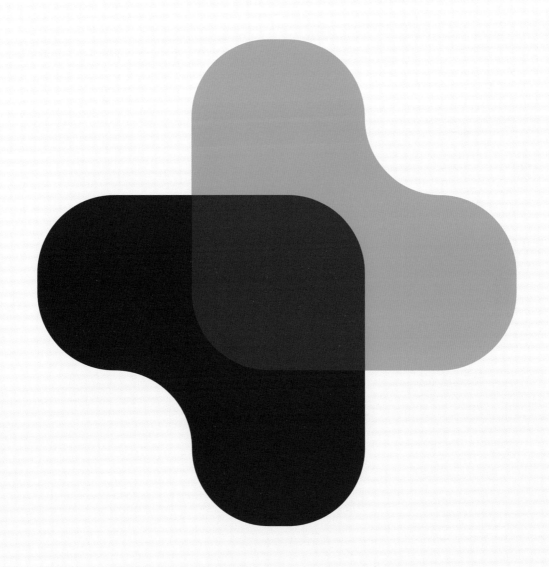

A.1 Prior to TSIM initiation

The Ohio River Health System ("Ohio River") is a network of 10 hospitals and over 100 ambulatory practice sites spanning multiple states. Ohio River has a history of being recognized for delivering high-quality care. In 2016, Ohio River began to pilot telehealth services in the neurology and pediatric service lines, with some success.

When the COVID-19 pandemic occurred in 2020, Ohio River's IT department was able to quickly deploy a simple video conferencing platform for its physicians. While Ohio River leadership was pleased with the initial effort, they soon realized that the implementation and current delivery of telehealth were very fractured. Even though the IT department deployed a specific video client, they found some physicians were using other non-HIPAA compliant platforms that were allowed during the public health emergency (PHE). In addition, the providers did not feel they were getting adequate IT and operational support to deliver care efficiently so patient visits were taking longer than normal. When some of the Ohio River clinics began to reopen, many providers struggled with how to smoothly deliver both in-person and telehealth care.

Ohio River was already planning to invest resources into expanding its telehealth infrastructure prior to the pandemic. During the PHE, Ohio River was awarded significant grant funding to match its planned investment into developing telehealth services to improve healthcare access for medically underserved areas.

With the known challenges that the system was facing and the financial investments being made, Ohio River leadership decided that its health system needed to centralize telehealth governance and support, and ensure its team had the education and training to successfully develop, implement, and sustain telehealth services. Ohio River sent four members of its team to be trained on TSIM. Ohio River primarily focused on IT aspects of telehealth service development and so the original team that completed TSIM training did not include a clinical champion or a staff member with expertise in existing clinical workflows. Additionally, because of the relaxation of various telehealth-related regulations due to the PHE, Ohio River had not focused on the telehealth privileging or malpractice issues for its providers and did not have telehealth sustainability plans in place. Fortunately, the telehealth prerequisite information incorporated into TSIM enabled them to develop the checklist below prior to embarking on expansion of telehealth services. Each item often necessitated numerous meetings with relevant stakeholders and the necessary expertise. While time-consuming, Ohio River realized this preliminary work was essential to ensure that when telehealth service development began, it would proceed with as few roadblocks as possible.

A.1.1 TSIM prerequisite checklist

1   Engage system IT and network expertise and map out information security and interoperability needs.

2   Develop technology selection criteria and processes through focusing on clinical use case, operational functionality, and technical requirements and a common evaluation tool.

3   Identify potential clinical areas of focus and related telehealth delivery mode.

4   Initiate preliminary discussions with major telehealth technology/software vendors.

5   Assess broadband capabilities in target communities/locations.

6   Develop a position description and hire a telehealth services manager/administrator; ideally this hire should have some background in finance and/or people management.

7   Identify and recruit a physician champion with institutional respect amongst the medical staff.

8   Engage system legal and regulatory expertise. Early activities include privileging medical staff to provide telehealth services in their areas of practice, and reviewing malpractice coverage and the potential need for expanded coverage. Additionally, learn state-specific requirements for establishing a patient-provider relationship and prescribing medication via telehealth.

9   Review patient consent for treatment policies/forms and revise if needed for telehealth.

10   Evaluate documentation issues and the electronic health record (EHR) for internal telehealth delivery and outward-facing telehealth delivery to sites not part of Ohio River.

11   Conduct fair market value assessment of Ohio River's telehealth services for pricing purposes.

12   Incorporate sustainability planning, including potential pathways for both return and value on investment.

13   Identify the key primary value drivers to develop telehealth services at Ohio River.

14   Collaborate with the compliance department to develop pathways for professional service and site of delivery billing to occur.

15   Apply National Quality Forum's Telehealth Measurement Framework for outcomes planning, including an early focus on utilization and patient-provider experience measurement.

16   Identify technical reliability metrics and sustainability metrics.

Once substantial progress had been made on the above prerequisites, including hiring a telehealth program manager and establishing an executive medical director, Ohio River solicited telehealth ideas from within its system. The following sections describe how it managed all of the new telehealth ideas using TSIM.

A.2 TSIM Pipeline and Strategy phases

After the initial surge of telehealth activity due to the pandemic, the Ohio River telehealth team began to regroup and organize. With news spreading that the organization was pushing forward with telehealth adoption and more resources being available, a flurry of telehealth ideas started to flood the telehealth department. Fortunately, a system was put in place to serve as the Pipeline and begin to collect pertinent data on each request. Some ideas were immediately identified as out of scope or not in line with the organization's vision (e.g.

international telehealth). For the other ideas, the telehealth team met with the requestors and used a standard intake form to begin to define the scope of the service idea and understand the problem that it was attempting to solve. The telehealth team began to consolidate around two main ideas – telestroke (contracted care value driver) and school-based telehealth (health equity value driver) – which were advanced through the Strategy phase. In order to guide the pace of program development, the telehealth team used the completed intake forms to score both service ideas using TSIM templates.

Next, metrics of success and potential sustainability business models were determined for each service. The team concluded that the telestroke service could be established and made sustainable with contractual revenue and professional billing. With a standardized approach across the system, the team would measure utilization and "door-to-needle" (DTN) times as core performance metrics. While there were initial concerns of sustainability for the school-based telehealth service, it addressed an Ohio River strategic imperative to improve pediatric care to medically underserved areas. In addition, the grant funding that Ohio River received was sufficient to cover the program's expenses while the Ohio River government relations team lobbied for improved payment policies. The school-based team would track utilization and total number of children with access to the program as core metrics. Tables A.1–A.5 illustrate how Ohio River utilized the TSIM intake and prioritization scoring tools for both programs.

A.2.1 TSIM intake form and TSIM prioritization score for telestroke

Ohio River has a very strong neurosciences program and a part of the clinical enterprise's strategic plan is to expand these services through telehealth. The problem being solved via telehealth is largely related to a lack of stroke neurologists in many smaller communities served by Ohio River and thus patients with acute stroke not receiving expert-directed care. Ohio River also stand to benefit as a health system through improved triage and transfer decision-making with regard to which patients with acute ischemic stroke are eligible for catheter-directed thrombectomy or need other advanced therapeutic interventions available only on its main campus.

A.2.2 TSIM intake form and TSIM prioritization score for school-based telehealth

Because a substantial portion of the external funding Ohio River received is intended to improve access to care for underserved communities, the planning team identified school-based telehealth as a second area of focus. The proposers plan to focus on providing both acute visits and chronic asthma management support to children in schools. The team submitting the intake form is highly engaged and committed to reducing health inequities among children in the Ohio River catchment area.

The telehealth team continued partnering with the telestroke and school-based telehealth clinical champions to identify appropriate performance metrics for both programs. Recognizing the uncertainty with regard to service demand and uptake, the group agreed to focus on short- and medium-term outcomes for the first year of each program. After the first year in Operations, plans were made to review performance metrics for possible inclusion of long-term outcomes. The initial performance metrics are outlined in Table A.5.

Table A.1 TSIM intake form for telestroke

Date	August 28, 2021
Telehealth service idea	Telestroke consultation for emergency departments
Service requestor	Tiffany Schroeder, VP of Neurology Services
Service line	Neurology
Who will be the executive champion?	Tiffany Schroeder, VP of Neurology Services
Who will be the clinical champion(s)?	Dr. Brooklyn Rae, Dr. Cecilia Rose, Dr. Scarlett Raine
Define the scope of the service	The telestroke service will evaluate patients presenting to emergency departments with suspected acute stroke for initial treatment recommendations
What problem is being solved via telehealth?	This service will improve access to expert stroke care that is limited or not available in many community hospitals
What condition(s) will be treated?	Acute ischemic stroke
When will the service be available?	24/7/365 given emergent nature of ischemic stroke
Who will be the consulting providers?	Stroke neurologists
Where will the patients be located?	Hospitals – emergency department
How will success of the service be measured?	Process of care measures (e.g. time to initial stroke evaluation, time to therapy); utilization; Net Promoter Score
What is the business model or pathway to sustainability?	Hospitals will be charged for access to the service; professional billing will be submitted for each encounter
What workflow will be used?	Emergent condition workflow
What telehealth modality will be used? Other technology requirements?	Real-time synchronous video encounters, delivered on a cart-based solution with pan-tilt-zoom (PTZ); telehealth software with image sharing
Expected primary value	Contracted care – hospital support service

Table A.2 TSIM prioritization score for telestroke

Category	Domain	Scoring criteria
Implementation support	Strategic alignment	(4) Addresses objectives/needs of the enterprise's strategic plan
		3) Addresses objectives/needs of the clinical department's strategic plan
		2) Considered priority of the clinical division
		1) Has clinical leadership's support
	Provider champion(s)	(4) Multiple providers engaged
		3) Single provider engaged
		2) Provider champion identified
		1) No provider champion identified
	Provider capacity	(4) Adequate capacity to implement and expand the service
		3) Adequate capacity to implement the service
		2) Adequate capacity to pilot the service
		1) Need to strategically hire to pilot the service
Potential impact	Total cost of care	4) Service is expected to have a significant reduction in total cost of care
		(3) Service is expected to have a moderate reduction in total cost of care
		2) Service is expected to have a minimal reduction in total cost of care
		1) Service is not expected to reduce the total cost of care
	Quality	(4) Service is projected to significantly improve quality outcomes
		3) Service is projected to have a moderate improvement in quality outcomes
		2) Service is projected to have a minimal improvement in quality outcomes
		1) Service is not projected to improve quality outcomes

Category	Domain	Scoring criteria
Potential impact, *continued*	Access to care	(4) Service is projected to significantly increase access to care for a target patient population
		3) Service is projected to make a moderate improvement for accessing care for the overall population
		2) Service is projected to make a slight improvement for accessing care
		1) Service is not expected to increase access to care
Sustainability	Potential market reach	4) Service has potential to serve a national market
		(3) Service has potential to serve a region of the national market
		2) Service has potential to serve the statewide population
		1) Service is likely to be limited to serving the local region
	Financial analysis	4) Proven business model with a significant ROI
		(3) New business model with a significant projected ROI
		2) Business model with a minimally/moderately projected ROI
		1) Business model has substantial sustainability risks
	Current demand	(4) Service is in high demand with patients and/or referring sites
		3) Service has moderate level of demand with patients and/or referring sites
		2) Service has interest expressed by potential patients and/or referring sites
		1) Interest/demand for service is unknown
Total priority score = 33		

Technology evaluation also continued at a brisk pace. Request for proposal (RFP) documents were distributed via Ohio River's procurement department and select telehealth technology vendors were approached to participate in the RFP process. Dual documentation and the capacity to "push" patient notes from the telehealth platform to a patient's EHR were considered high priorities. The telehealth solutions embedded in Ohio River's EHR were quickly discarded as these were highly complex and required patient-created accounts; thus they were not amenable to urgent patient evaluations or to supporting patients who were not already part of Ohio River. Technology evaluation was started and continued during the Development phase. The goal was to have the new telehealth services live within six months. After charters were created to outline allocated resources and clearly define the scope of each telehealth service, they were signed by the leadership of the telehealth team and the requesting clinical departments.

Table A.3 TSIM intake form for school-based telehealth

Date	August 28, 2021
Telehealth service idea	School-based telehealth
Service requestor	Jacklyn Martin, MD – Chair General Pediatrics
Service line	Children's services
Who will be the executive champion?	Don Harley, MBA – Administrator for Pediatrics
Who will be the clinical champion(s)?	Deb Reynolds, MD; Ron Deere, RN
Define the scope of the service	School-based telehealth will be delivered from Ohio River general pediatrics department to school nurse offices to provide both acute evaluations (e.g. earache) as well as acute and chronic asthma management
What problem is being solved via telehealth?	Some counties lack pediatric care; children missing school to be evaluated in local emergency departments for minor problems; no pathway for asthma medication administration in schools as no local providers
What condition(s) will be treated?	Acute pediatric conditions, chronic asthma care
When will the service be available?	On demand and scheduled during school hours
Who will be the consulting providers?	Pediatricians and pediatric advanced practice providers
Where will the patients be located?	School nurse offices
How will success of the service be measured?	Process of care measures (e.g. adherence to asthma controller medications); utilization; Net Promoter Score
What is the business model or pathway to sustainability?	Advocacy to get schools designated as a Medicaid site of care; professional billing will be submitted for each encounter; external funding
What workflow will be used?	On-demand workflow; scheduled encounter workflow
What telehealth modality will be used? Other technology requirements?	Real-time synchronous video encounters, delivered on a cart-based solution with pan-tilt-zoom (PTZ); carts equipped with peripheral devices (e.g. otoscope, stethoscope)
Expected primary value	Health equity

Table A.4 TSIM prioritization score for school-based telehealth

Category	Domain	Scoring criteria
Implementation support	Strategic alignment	(4) Addresses objectives/needs of the enterprise's strategic plan
		3) Addresses objectives/needs of the clinical department's strategic plan
		2) Considered priority of the clinical division
		1) Has clinical leadership's support
	Provider champion(s)	(4) Multiple providers engaged
		3) Single provider engaged
		2) Provider champion identified
		1) No provider champion identified
	Provider capacity	4) Adequate capacity to implement and expand the service
		(3) Adequate capacity to implement the service
		2) Adequate capacity to pilot the service
		1) Need to strategically hire to pilot the service
Potential impact	Total cost of care	(4) Service is expected to have a significant reduction in total cost of care
		3) Service is expected to have a moderate reduction in total cost of care
		2) Service is expected to have a minimal reduction in total cost of care
		1) Service is not expected to reduce the total cost of care
	Quality	(4) Service is projected to significantly improve quality outcomes
		3) Service is projected to have a moderate improvement in quality outcomes
		2) Service is projected to have a minimal improvement in quality outcomes
		1) Service is not projected to improve quality outcomes

Table continues

Table A.4 continued

Category	Domain	Scoring criteria
Potential impact, *continued*	Access to care	(4) Service is projected to significantly increase access to care for a target patient population
		3) Service is projected to make a moderate improvement for accessing care for the overall population
		2) Service is projected to make a slight improvement for accessing care
		1) Service is not expected to increase access to care
Sustainability	Potential market	4) Service has potential to serve a national market
		3) Service has potential to serve a region of the national market
		(2) Service has potential to serve the statewide population
		1) Service is likely to be limited to serving the local region
	Financial analysis	4) Proven business model with a significant ROI
		3) New business model with a significant projected ROI
		2) Business model with a minimally/moderately projected ROI
		(1) Business model has substantial sustainability risks
	Current demand	4) Service is in high demand with patients and/or referring sites
		(3) Service has moderate level of demand with patients and/or referring sites
		2) Service has interest expressed by potential patients and/or referring sites
		1) Interest/demand for service is unknown
Total priority score = 29		

Table A.5 Performance metrics for telestroke and school-based telehealth

Metric	Measure
Utilization	Number of telestroke consults requested and completed
	Number of children evaluated via telehealth for acute problems and chronic disease management
Provider experience	Net Promoter Score from providers (obtain both telehealth provider and referring providers)
Patient experience	Net Promoter Score from patients/parents
Quality of care	DTN time for patients with acute ischemic stroke seen via telehealth; increased use of asthma controller medications for children seen via telehealth
Reliability	Ratio of "dropped" telehealth visits relative to completed visits
Sustainability	Contracted payments cover cost for telestroke program within one year of program inception; state Medicaid plan revises coverage policy to include schools as a site of care

A.3 TSIM Development phase

Because of TSIM training, the Ohio River teams realized Development would be the most complex and time-consuming phase. The telehealth program manager was selected because of her extensive experience in complex project management and ability to work with multiple stakeholder groups to achieve consensus. These skills would prove essential over the next six months. The program manager established and guided working groups focused on each of the four major pathways in Development: (1) clinical, (2) technology, (3) legal and regulatory, and (4) outcomes. Prior to launching the working groups, the telehealth program manager organized a 90-minute pre-check meeting that included representation from the clinical champions, informatics, IT, legal, billing compliance, revenue cycle, scheduling, credentialing, risk management, information security, and procurement. During the pre-check meeting, the telehealth service charters were briefly reviewed and the driving questions for each pathway discussed at a high level. Additionally, stakeholders were oriented to the RACI matrix so that members understood that for different tasks and deliverables they might be either responsible, accountable, consulted, or informed. This served to manage expectations and also establish that a clear owner would be assigned for the work ahead. It was determined that the working groups would meet concurrently and intersect as needed, and each group established a series of recurring meetings at a brisk cadence to meet the target six-month timeline. Sections A.3.1–A.3.4 explore the activities of each pathway working group in more detail.

A.3.1 TSIM Development: clinical pathway

Developing a robust clinical workflow is one of the most important elements of TSIM. Without a systematic and organized approach to how, when, and where the patient will be connected with the remote provider, the telehealth service will fail – largely through provider and/or patient disengagement. The driving questions in developing the clinical pathway include:

1   What is the ideal clinical workflow of the telehealth service?
2   What system development and/or configurations are needed to support the clinical workflow?
3   What type of scheduling support is required to support the service?
4   What training will be required and what educational/training resources need to be created?

In order to understand how the new telehealth workflows would integrate with the provider's existing workflows, the telehealth program manager spent several days shadowing the stroke neurologists as they responded to institutional brain attacks in Ohio River's emergency department and similarly shadowed the general pediatricians. It became readily apparent that the clinical workflows for the two new services would be quite different due to differences in patient acuity, location, and service demand. The telestroke service would require a 24/7 on-demand workflow. The school-based telehealth service would need a scheduled workflow for chronic condition management as well as an on-demand workflow for acute issues. The first step in establishing the clinical pathway was to develop high-level swim lane diagrams (see Figures A.1–A.3).

A.3.1.1 Clinical pathway: telestroke

Using the swim lane diagrams as a starting point, the clinical teams began mapping other key operational considerations. For telestroke, it was determined that most patients would be transferred to Ohio River's main campus after receiving thrombolysis. This was deemed important for patient safety as the referring hospitals lacked experience in monitoring for post-thrombolytic complications. However, longer-term planning and implementation would focus on developing protocols with the referring hospitals, combined with teleneurology follow-up support, so that patients could remain in their local hospital in the future.

The telestroke clinical team adapted Ohio River protocols and training materials to the partner hospital's resources and substantial focus was placed on training in stroke recognition. The clinical champions also wanted to ensure that the local emergency medical services were trained in acute stroke recognition so that the emergency department would be alerted prior to the patient's actual arrival. The referring hospitals agreed contractually to a monthly on-call telestroke fee that was tiered based on each hospital's overall emergency department volumes. A daily on-call schedule was developed with the stroke neurologists that included both a primary on-call physician and a backup physician in case the primary neurologist was already engaged in a telehealth consult when another activation call came in through the Ohio River access center.

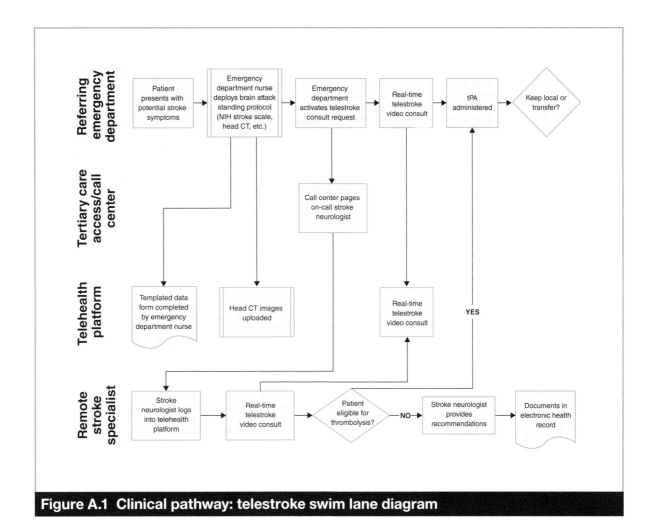

Figure A.1 Clinical pathway: telestroke swim lane diagram

Training materials included content related to telehealth technology use, criteria for telestroke consult activation, training in how to perform National Institutes of Health (NIH) stroke scale assessments, and overall stroke education. Communication protocols were developed between Ohio River and the partner hospitals, including estimated response times once a telestroke consult request had been made to the access center. Training also emphasized that this program was focused on potential acute stroke evaluation and management and not on more general neurological issues seen in the emergency department.

A.3.1.2 Clinical pathway: school-based telehealth

The clinical workflow for school-based telehealth included both scheduled and on-demand pathways. Because the service would only be offered during school hours, it was determined that telehealth support would not extend to after-school, weekends, or holidays. The program's clinical champions, after reviewing local epidemiological data, reported that there was a compelling need for improved asthma management in the initial targeted counties. In fact, two of the counties had rates of emergency department visits for pediatric asthma four times higher than the overall region. Thus, a workflow for routine asthma evaluation and management was

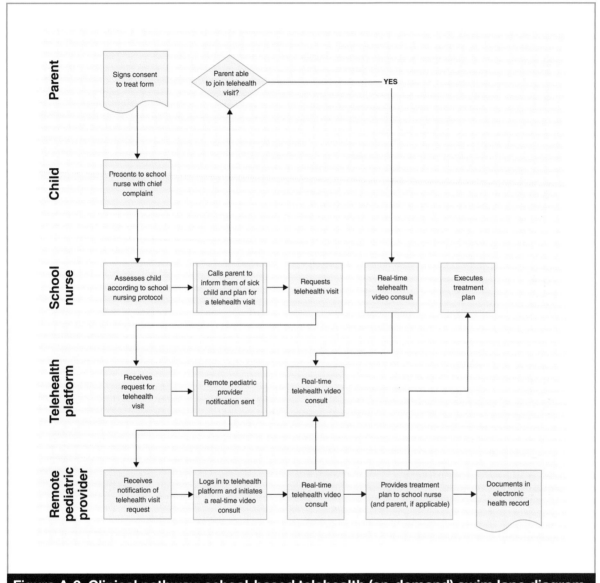

Figure A.2 Clinical pathway: school-based telehealth (on-demand) swim lane diagram

initiated and grounded in the NIH's Asthma Action Plan's best-practice recommendations. This included child and parent asthma education, child inhaler technique coaching, and medication management offered between the school nurse and the remote prescribing provider. The plan was to have parents sign consent forms prior to their children being treated in the program and they could participate in the scheduled visits remotely if they desired. The need for a three-way video conferencing ability was deemed a key feature and passed along to the technology pathway working group. The school nurse worked with Ohio River's access center to coordinate appointments for scheduled asthma care visits with physicians, respiratory therapists, and asthma educators. Additionally, a workflow was created for acute pediatric issues such as earache and other common acute ailments of childhood.

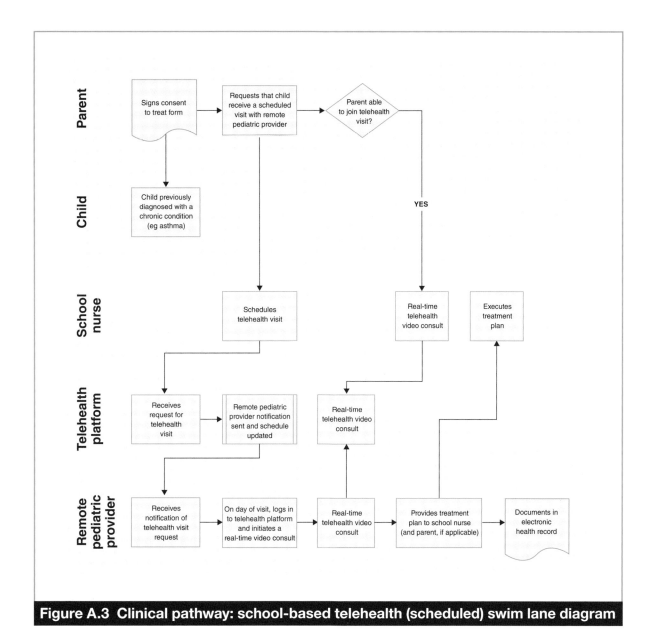

Figure A.3 Clinical pathway: school-based telehealth (scheduled) swim lane diagram

The clinical champions recognized the importance of preserving the patient's medical home where possible and so they developed on-demand workflows that included local pediatric and primary care practices as well as pediatric nurse practitioners working in Ohio River's main campus. The telehealth platform was programmed with first, second, and third call pathways and, based on the preferences of local primary care providers, the local providers could either serve in one of these call positions or opt out altogether, in which case Ohio River's nurse practitioners would manage the acute call. Thus, the telehealth platform needed to enable a call tree approach to activation, and this requirement was provided to the technology working group.

Training materials focused heavily on the school nurses as this group would be the primary point of access between schoolchildren and the telehealth team. The clinical champions and telehealth program manager made several visits to school-based health clinics to better understand the on-site workflows of school nurses and quickly ascertained that this group of nurses had extremely busy schedules and that insertion of telehealth could easily become an added burden without excellent service from the telehealth program. Additionally, it was quickly determined that very user-friendly and simple-to-activate technology would be instrumental to the program's success as there was substantial variation in the technology savviness of school nurses. Finally, clinical training for the school nurses focused on chronic asthma management and, to a lesser degree, pediatric mental health as this clinical focus appeared a likely second phase for the program based on perceived needs amongst school administrators.

A.3.2 TSIM Development: technology pathway

Initial technology considerations were undertaken as part of Ohio River's pre-TSIM planning efforts and thus the telehealth team had a general idea of the telehealth platform options available. The team had also undertaken an assessment of broadband availability in the initial target communities. Fortunately, all acute care hospitals in the state had adequate broadband access due to a prior program sponsored by the Federal Communication Commission to ensure ubiquitous broadband in US acute care hospitals. Similarly, schools in the target communities generally had broadband access. The connectivity limitations were mostly related to internal infrastructure deficiencies within a subset of hospitals and schools. Because this had been identified previously, these sites were able to start making infrastructure investments to improve wireless access internal to their facilities. Ohio River decided that its IT departments would partner with their IT peers at partner sites to install and test the telehealth platforms and that 24/7 IT help desk support would need to be included as part of telehealth vendor contracts. Program-specific technology pathways are outlined below.

A.3.2.1 Technology pathway: telestroke

The clinical needs dictated the technology choices for telestroke, and major selection criteria included the ability to conduct real-time, two-way audio-visual consultations, to upload radiographic images for viewing by the remote stroke expert, and to "push" documentation from the telehealth platform into partner hospitals' EHRs. The need for cart or other mobile solutions was also evident as the telehealth platform would be moved to different locations when partnering emergency departments based on where patients were located. Value-added technology features included templated clinical intake forms that could be completed quickly by the bedside emergency department nurse and time-based prompts to optimize timely assessment and treatment for acute ischemic stroke.

A.3.2.2 Technology pathway: school-based telehealth

Because the school-based telehealth program planned to rely on school nurses to access patients, it was clear that a "plug and play" technology option would better enable program uptake due to ease of use. Additionally, the clinical champions determined that physical examination peripheral accessories were necessary to perform assessments such as chest auscultation and inner ear examination. Also, the telehealth platform needed to have call tree functionality to escalate acute care needs and the ability for three-way audio-visual communication so visits could be arranged between the school/child, remote provider, and the child's caregivers. Finally, the platform would need easy-to-access documentation tools that were compliant with both HIPAA and FERPA (Family Educational Rights and Privacy Act) regulations, and the ability to push reports to the school health records and EHRs of local providers when relevant.

A.3.3 TSIM Development: legal and regulatory pathway

The legal and compliance departments had been engaged during the early planning stages for telehealth services and completed a review of Ohio River's credentialing bylaws and malpractice coverage. It was determined that medical staff would have provision of care via telehealth in their area of practice added to their list of privileges. The patient consent for treatment documentation was adapted for care delivered via telehealth. The working group for this pathway then focused on service-specific legal and regulatory issues, including details specific to the planned services, impact on providers, and contracting with partner sites.

It was determined that Ohio River stroke specialists needed to obtain privileges at partner hospitals when the hospital was not part of Ohio River, and the medical staff office assigned a team member to be responsible for this effort. The business model for telestroke necessitated a fair market value assessment of the service, as Ohio River would be charging partner hospitals for this support. School-based telehealth was not planning to charge schools for services but did plan to submit professional fee charges, and thus the compliance department worked to ensure adherence to third-party payor policies. Finally, both hospitals and schools signed contracts with Ohio River that stipulated the roles and responsibilities of each site and outlined precisely how support would be provided and what the partner site would provide with regard to financial, personnel, and other support needed for the program.

A.3.4 TSIM Development: outcomes pathway

During the Strategy phase outcomes had been mapped out for each program and now the working group focused on potential data sources, data collection, and data reporting. The working groups mapped out a plan for outcomes collection as shown in Tables A.6 and A.7.

After much discussion and planning through the journey of the Development pathways, it was time to hold the launch status brief. After all decisions were reviewed it was determined that while there were several outstanding elements related to vendor contracts and timelines for provider credentialing, the team was ready to move the projects forward into the Implementation phase.

Table A.6 Telestroke outcomes assessment

Outcome category	Metric	Data source	Data validation	Data reporting
Utilization	Number of telestroke interactions	Data extraction from telehealth platform and call center	Reconcile data between the two sources	Weekly for telestroke team; monthly for external hospitals; quarterly for Ohio River leadership
Provider experience	Net Promoter Score	Secure electronic survey tool distributed via email	Qualitative interviews with referring and consulting providers	Monthly for telestroke team and external hospitals; annually for Ohio River leadership
Patient experience	Net Promoter Score	Secure electronic survey tool distributed via email	Qualitative interviews with patients/families	Monthly for telestroke team and external hospitals; annually for Ohio River leadership
Quality of care	DTN time	Telehealth platform	Review sample of patient records; reconcile	Weekly for telestroke team; monthly for external hospitals; quarterly for Ohio River leadership
Reliability	Ratio of dropped to completed visits	Telehealth platform	Track for consistency over time; vendor IT help desk requests	Weekly for telestroke team; monthly for telehealth platform vendor
Sustainability	Combined revenue from hospital contract + professional fee collection	Accounting and financial management systems; billing data extraction	Reconcile observed vs. predicted revenues	Monthly for telestroke team; annually for Ohio River leadership

Table A.7 School-based telehealth outcomes assessment

Outcome category	Metric	Data source	Data validation	Data reporting
Utilization	Number of school-based telehealth interactions	Data extraction from telehealth platform and call center	Reconcile data between the two sources	Weekly for school-based team; monthly for external partners; quarterly for Ohio River leadership
Provider experience	Net Promoter Score	Secure electronic survey tool distributed via email	Qualitative interviews with referring and consulting providers	Monthly for school-based team and external partners; annually for Ohio River leadership
Patient experience	Net Promoter Score	Secure electronic survey tool distributed via email	Qualitative interviews with patients/families	Monthly for school-based team and external partners; annually for Ohio River leadership
Quality of care	Adherence to asthma controller medications	EHR; pharmacy system	Review sample of patient records; reconcile	Weekly for school-based team; monthly for external partners; quarterly for Ohio River leadership
Reliability	Ratio of dropped to completed visits	Telehealth platform	Track for consistency over time; vendor IT help desk requests	Weekly for school-based team; monthly for telehealth platform vendor
Sustainability	Medicaid professional billing revenue	Billing data extraction	Reconcile observed vs. predicted revenues	Monthly for school-based team; annually for Ohio River leadership

A.4 TSIM Implementation phase

It is an exciting time at Ohio River, in which the actual implementation of the chosen telehealth programs is to begin. Roundtable discussions are arranged for both programs, bringing the support teams and the providers together to talk about the workflows that have been developed and to discuss the reasonings for them. They discuss the training elements that are needed and how the providers will be supported as they begin to do clinical work in this new way.

After the roundtables, training and mock calls are scheduled and the providers get hands-on experience going through the workflow and connecting with the technologies. Competency assessments are done for the providers and supporting staff, which provide a sense of security for the team members. Next, the team goes through a pre-go-live procedure in which they double check that all the core elements of the infrastructure are working as intended. The video endpoints are all deemed in place and operational, the EHR templates are configured and available to providers, and the billing routing is determined to be accurate. The team declares that both the telestroke and school-based health programs have the all-clear to proceed with go-live.

The telestroke program hits the ground running, as on the first morning of go-live, a potential stroke patient is being seen at a nearby community hospital and the telestroke workflow is activated. From this first consult several opportunities to reinforce the workflow are identified and the telehealth support team stays involved throughout the process. The patient receives the recommended therapy within the target timeframe, and the team celebrates success. By the time a post-go-live debrief is scheduled (see Table A.8), several more telestroke consults have been conducted and a recurring theme of a need to reinforce the designed workflow with additional education and training becomes apparent as one partner hospital continues to activate telestroke consultation for an array of non-stroke neurological symptoms.

The school-based telehealth program has a scheduled visit on the day of go-live, which goes well, and the parent of the child expresses gratitude for her child not missing a day of school. Two weeks pass before the next visit; an on-demand consult occurs, and several more phone calls than predicted are needed to arrange the visit via the initial workflow. At the post-go-live debrief (see Table A.9) the team discusses plans for continued engagement, interval training for the providers and referring school nurses, and the need to establish plans for increased utilization.

Table A.8 Telestroke post-go-live debrief checklist

Checklist item	Status
Utilization	Visits are occurring in higher numbers than anticipated, with a number of "false alarms" or non-stroke consults
Documentation and billing audit	Billing charges and documentation appropriate, with some providers needing reminders to complete notes in a timely manner
Patient and provider experience	Verbal feedback from providers and patients is highly supportive; surveys pending
Service success	The service is considered a great success, although concerns about volume of consults versus staffing are raised
Operations phase entry	A number of improvements are recommended to the workflow and additional collaborations between consulting and referring teams are planned. The team anticipates moving the program to the Operations phase

Table A.9 School-based telehealth post-go-live debrief checklist

Checklist item	Status
Utilization	Visits are occurring as anticipated, although it is clear an engagement plan will be needed to meet the anticipated utilization targets
Documentation and billing audit	No concerns raised with documentation and billing compliance audit
Patient and provider experience	Verbal feedback from providers and patients is extremely supportive. School nurses express some concerns over time commitment and request referral efficiency improvements
Service success	The service is considered successful from an individual patient perspective. The need to target chronic disease conditions in order to demonstrate outcomes in the longer term is discussed
Operations phase entry	A number of workflow edits to accommodate the needs of the school nurse are discussed, as is the need to reinforce training on the workflow until volumes increase. The team feels that the program should remain in the Implementation phase while the planned changes are introduced

A.5 TSIM Operations phase

Within three months of the initial go-live, both of Ohio River's new telehealth programs have moved into the Operations phase of TSIM. In order to maintain and mature the clinical operations that have been established with these programs, oversight mechanisms are put in place that include a mixture of unique governance committees and assimilation into existing processes at Ohio River. The oversight structure seeks to guide and address the operational domains of service delivery management and operational technology management.

A.5.1 TSIM Operations: service delivery management

A.5.1.1 Telestroke

With predictable volumes now occurring with the telestroke program, Ohio River's attention turns to maturing the management of an enduring service. Following the TSIM framework, a service delivery management structure is put in place to assist with the engagement of people, hardwiring the process, and managing performance. For telestroke, quarterly check-ins with partnering hospitals are centered around feedback from the teams involved and a review of DTN times, compared with peer hospitals. A regular telestroke report and discussion are embedded into the Ohio River's neurology department medical staff meeting, which includes a review of provider productivity and the financial impact of the program. A steering committee is formed to include support staff and the designated clinical champion to continually work on program optimizations. Finally, an annual report to insurance payors is planned to encourage maintenance and further growth of telehealth-friendly reimbursement policies. Figure A.4 shows the number of telestroke consultations by month.

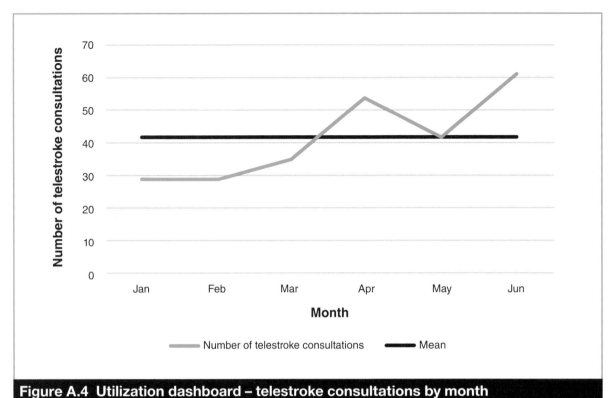

Figure A.4 Utilization dashboard – telestroke consultations by month

Several optimizations are changed at the telestroke steering committee in order to address process and performance management elements. The previously developed competency processes for providers and support staff are embedded in employee onboarding procedures and assigned as annual competencies for participating individuals. Special attention is paid to readiness for the Joint Commission review, including preparation for adding unique telestroke elements into the Ongoing Professional Practice Evaluation.

The telestroke software fortunately provides a unique set of process metrics that allow for report generation on the speed (e.g. time to consult, time to thrombolytic administration) and disposition of patients (e.g. proportion transferred, hemorrhagic bleed rates, rehab admission and survival). These metrics are leveraged for regular process reporting at the steering committee. The Ohio River patient safety oversight governance is also engaged, and an agreement is made to include incident discussion and action through those mechanisms, with outreach for inclusion of the partnering site as necessary. The monthly performance reports continue to demonstrate favorable Net Promoter Scores, a positive net profit margin, and strong technical reliability of the telestroke network. Unfortunately, the quality of care metric (i.e. DTN times) is not achieving the "60 minutes or less" goal across the telestroke network (see Figure A.5).

A.5.1.2 School-based telehealth

As the school-based telehealth team plans continued growth with partnering school districts, effort is made to continue to hardwire best-practice workflows and maintain consistent engagement with the people involved. For school-based care, this is a diverse

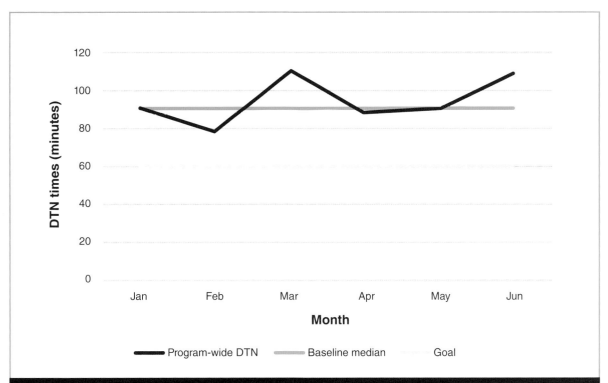

Figure A.5 Quality of care delivery dashboard – telestroke average DTN times by month

set of stakeholders in addition to the internal team, which includes school nurses, school administrators, school-district leadership, parent associations, and the school wellness oversight committee. Payors and local philanthropy are also part of the sustainability plan for the Ohio River program. It is important for Ohio River to maintain strong relationships with independent local primary care providers. In order to manage this complex set of stakeholders, an external-facing reporting and advisory committee structure is established. Monthly newsletters are designed, and an annual performance report is planned to include utilization per school population and percent of school population enrolled. A sustainability update will be included in the report that shows a pie chart representing the program's funding portfolio relative to the operating costs of the program. Figure A.6 shows the number of school-based telehealth consultations by month.

While utilization remains low, the monthly performance reports demonstrate a positive growth trend. For the internal team supporting school-based telehealth at Ohio River, the initial experience highlights that the unique needs of each child served and the characteristics of the school engaged require a regular cadence of communication. A scheduled review of utilization and quality of care delivery metrics occurs in the pediatric department's monthly medical staff meeting, and a weekly school-based telehealth team meeting is established. The support team expands to include a family patient liaison and social worker in order to assist with the management of any caregiver concerns that are generated during the course of clinical care and case management. The assigned billing compliance managers are engaged to ensure an adequate sample size for provider billing audits, and a monthly report that reviews reimbursement revenues is established.

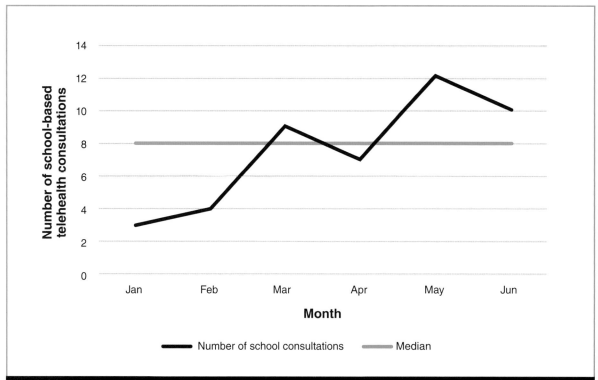

Figure A.6 Utilization dashboard – school-based telehealth consultations by month

A.5.2 TSIM Operations: operational technology management

While the telestroke and school-based telehealth programs have differing technology needs, the decision is made at Ohio River to maintain a centralized core IT support team for telehealth operations. A primary point of contact is assigned on the IT team for regular communications with the telestroke software vendor, and a larger team is cross-trained for support of video endpoints and troubleshooting. While an incident management system was originally integrated with the IT help desk during Development, the telehealth team identifies that the traditional Ohio River technical support does not always possess the telehealth technology expertise required to rapidly troubleshoot issues when patient care is immediately impacted. A core rapid response telehealth team is formed, and a new operational technology management workflow is created to triage calls appropriately. In addition, a system of tracking the expanding list of video endpoints and checking on the operational status of these endpoints at regular intervals is put in place. A reporting structure is created to monitor video and audio quality, technical failure rates, and the overall reliability of the video network. Lastly, a management process for planned system downtimes and a communication mechanism for unplanned downtimes are proactively put in place. Figure A.7 summarizes Ohio River's IT support process.

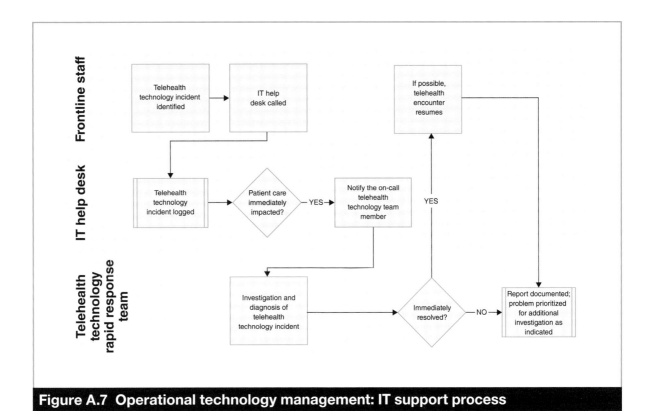

Figure A.7 Operational technology management: IT support process

A.6 TSIM Continuous Quality Improvement

Initially, Ohio River struggled with accessing accurate and timely telehealth data. The data collection and management processes were extremely manual, with each program maintaining its own Excel spreadsheets or Access databases. In some cases, even what was initially considered a simple utilization measure proved difficult to collect. The school-based telehealth program had to refer to the schedule each month and manually count how many telehealth visits occurred. The senior health system leadership grew frustrated with the inability to receive timely updates on telehealth utilization and without reliable data, managers were unable to monitor quality assurance or assess quality improvement interventions. To systematically address the data issues, the telehealth administrative leader created an interprofessional workgroup, known as the Continuous Quality Improvement (CQI) team, made up of stakeholders from the telehealth programs and informatics, and quality improvement personnel. The goal of this group was to standardize measure definitions and create a process for telehealth data to be automatically exported from the clinical data warehouse into dashboards for monitoring and identifying areas for improvement.

Now that the team has a systematic method for collecting and examining data, they can monitor for deviations from established program goals. The CQI team and leadership note the telestroke program's growth and continue to monitor telestroke utilization, but they identify the DTN time process measure as an area for improvement, as it is consistently higher than the 60-minute goal. The team takes a deeper dive into the DTN time data and determines that there is considerable variation across the rural telestroke hospitals. Going forward, rural telestroke hospitals are provided with a monthly report showing the hospital-specific DTN times, the median telestroke network DTN time, and the 60-minute goal as a benchmark. Telestroke coordinators in each location are instructed on how to interpret quality improvement run and control charts. Through this sub-analysis of the data, Baden Hilltop Hospital is identified as an outlier with DTN times frequently higher than the other telestroke hospitals (see Figure A.8). The CQI team initiates a service optimization request.

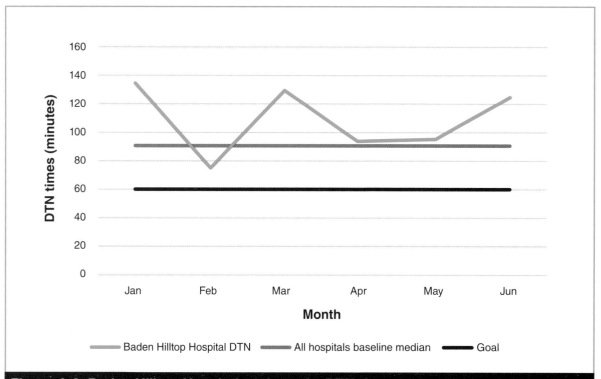

Figure A.8 Baden Hilltop Hospital – telestroke DTN times by month

Next, the CQI team works on a root cause analysis with emergency department leaders from Baden Hilltop Hospital to assess workflow adherence and interviews staff to identify barriers. Through collaborative CQI sessions, a fishbone diagram is drafted to identify potential causes of the longer DTN times. Findings from the root cause analysis include resistance by nurses to initiate the telestroke consultation, delays in getting tissue plasminogen activator (tPA) from the pharmacy, issues in staffing a full-time stroke coordinator, and delays in getting head CT scans. Figure A.9 provides the team's initial draft of a fishbone diagram.

The CQI team and Baden Hilltop Hospital emergency department leaders identify the delay in getting tPA from the pharmacy as the primary cause for poor DTN times. They focus on improving this process through Plan-Do-Study-Act (PDSA) cycles before investigating other secondary causes. After several rounds of the PDSA cycle, the team standardizes the workflow. The CQI team then begin working with other telestroke hospitals and repeat the PDSA process to improve DTN times.

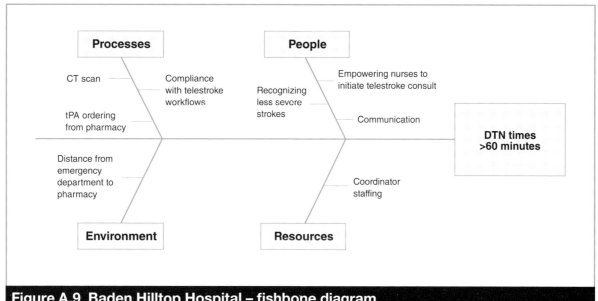

Figure A.9 Baden Hilltop Hospital – fishbone diagram

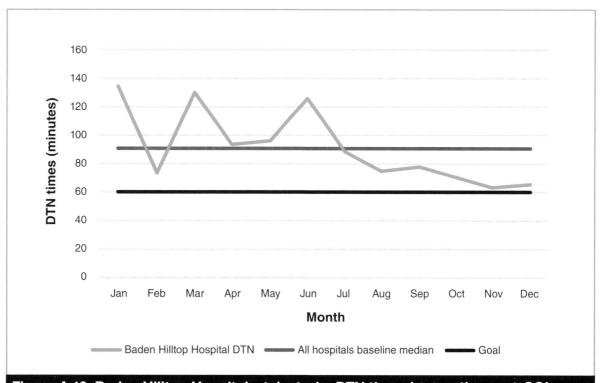

Figure A.10 Baden Hilltop Hospital – telestroke DTN times by month – post-CQI

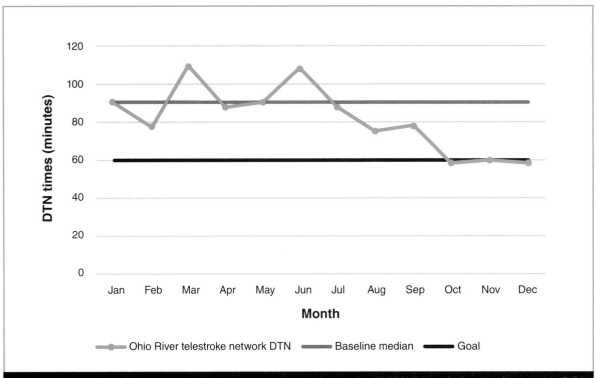

Figure A.11 Ohio River's telestroke network – telestroke DTN times by month – post-CQI

After the initial rounds of PDSA cycles, the CQI team is pleased with the improvements in DTN times. Baden Hilltop Hospital continues to improve its DTN times and is getting closer to the 60-minute goal (Figure A.10). The run chart now indicates a shift in performance. The telestroke hospitals are following the standard workflows, and the overall DTN times for Ohio River's telestroke network have met the 60-minute goal consistently over the last quarter (Figure A.11).

A.7 Ohio River case summary

Ohio River is now well established in its organizational telehealth journey. The program champions continue to be highly engaged, because they are seeing tangible outcomes in patient care associated with all the time and effort invested in applying TSIM to develop their respective programs. The mission-critical importance of developing and adhering to a clear strategy early in TSIM became apparent over time and helped avoid mission creep and other distractions so that Ohio River could maintain focus on its intended priorities. While the Development phase was time-consuming and sometimes tedious, troubleshooting issues as they arose and having a clear responsibility matrix allowed the teams to work through challenges. Overall the Implementation phase went smoothly and both telestroke and school-based telehealth transitioned quickly into Operations. CQI remains active and ongoing as the teams track outcomes and other metrics.

Index

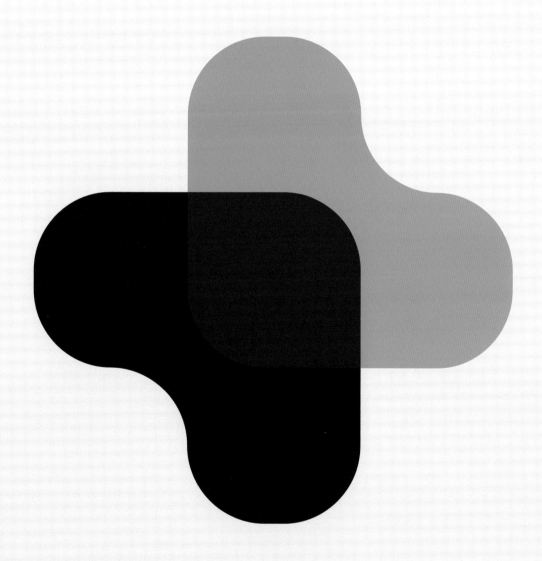

Index

Bold page numbers indicate figures, *italic* numbers indicate tables.